# MICRONUTRITION

## *for the Weight Loss Surgery Patient*

BY JACQUELINE JACQUES, ND

MATRIX MEDICAL COMMUNICATIONS

*Micronutrition for the Weight Loss Surgery Patient*
by Jacqueline Jacques, ND

Copyright © 2006 Matrix Medical Communications

*Publisher contact information:*

Matrix Medical Communications
4975 West Chester Pike
Suite 201
PO Box 445
Edgemont, PA 19028-0445
Phone: (610) 325-9905
Fax: (610) 325-9906
www.bariatrictimes.com

President/Group Publisher: Robert L. Dougherty
Partner: Patrick Scullin
Executive Editor: Elizabeth A. Klumpp
Managing Editor: Colleen M. Hutchinson
National Sales Manager: J. Gregory Francis

Printed in the United States.

ISBN 0-9768526-2-4

**Note from the publisher:** *This book provides basic information about a broad range of medical conditions. It is not intended to serve as a tool for diagnosing illness, in prescribing treatments, or as a substitute for the physician/patient relationship. All persons concerned about medical symptoms or the possibility of disease are encouraged to seek professional care from an appropriate healthcare provider.*

# Dedication

*T*his book could not have been accomplished without the support and encouragement of many people: Tom Kinder for bringing me to bariatrics; my family for putting up with me during the many weeks I stayed up very late at night writing; the countless bariatric health professionals who encouraged me (knowingly or not) with their questions and insights; and Matrix Medical Communications for helping to make this book a reality. Finally, and most importantly, this book is dedicated to the thousands of weight loss surgery patients for whom this book was ultimately written. Over the years, many of these patients have requested that this information be brought to their doctors, dietitians, and other caregivers, and this was the greatest motivation for the creation of this book.

*If taking vitamins doesn't keep you healthy enough, try more laughter: The most wasted of all days is that on which one has not laughed.*

—Sebastien Roch Nicolas Chamfort, 1741–1794
*French writer, journalist, and playwright*

# Table of Contents

# PART 3: PUTTING IT ALL TOGETHER

# PART 4: APPENDICES

# Foreword

*"I will apply dietetic measures for the benefit of the sick according to my ability and judgment; I will keep them from harm and injustice."*

**—Hippocrates**

*"I will prevent disease whenever I can, for prevention is preferable to cure."*

**—Dr. Louis Lasagna, 1964**
**Academic Dean**
**School of Medicine**
**Tufts University**

While surgery for the treatment of severe obesity was barely spoken about a decade ago, it now assumes an increasingly prominent role in the pursuit of normalized body weight and improved health. The fact is that in 2005, more than 170,000 bariatric procedures were performed in the United States, nearly a 10-fold increase since 1993. As sophistication in the field continues to grow, so does the need for evidence-based practice guidelines for nutritional management of the bariatric patient, specifically in the area of micronutrition.

In 1993, I joined a surgical practice that performed just a few bariatric cases a year, all restrictive procedures performed through an open approach. There existed only one textbook on obesity surgery, and a literature search would typically reveal just a handful of articles describing the rare case of a severe micronutrient deficiency. Those of us caring for bariatric surgery patients struggled to understand the nutritional needs of our patients and grappled with providing them sound advice on nutritional supplementation.

In writing this book, noted naturopathic practitioner Dr. Jacqueline Jacques brings together for the first time in one volume sound science-based information on the prevention, diagnosis, and treatment of micronutritional disorders. She has successfully developed a practical text that takes account of the best scientific evidence available. Dr. Jacques provides detailed and amplified information on a complex topic in a simple and practical manner. This concise guide makes a significant contribution to the continuing efforts of the bariatric community to improve the micronutritional status of their patients.

As practitioners treating the chronic disease of obesity, we are exhorted to model healthy lifestyles for our patients. It is our responsibility to monitor our patients and protect them from surgically induced malnutritive states. In this text, Dr. Jacques synthesizes and summarizes complex nutritional science in such a way so that the bariatric practitioner will be able to provide their patients with an opportunity for optimal health and longevity. This is a remarkable effort in a much needed area, which will benefit all who are striving to provide such care to their patients.

**Dory Roedel Ferraro, MS, CS, ANP**
*Assistant Professor of Clinical Nursing*
*Columbia University*
*Clinical Director, Center for Advanced Surgery*
*Lawrence Hospital Center*

# Introduction

As the challenge of obesity continues to affect the health of a growing number of Americans, those who opt to undergo weight loss surgery (WLS) are growing in number. According to the American Obesity Association, approximately 127 million adults in the US are overweight, 60 million are obese, and 9 million are morbidly obese. Moreover, we have every indication that these numbers are only increasing, with no immediate improvement in sight. To qualify for WLS, a patient must be morbidly obese (body mass index [BMI] of 40 or greater) or have a BMI of 35 to 40 with significant comorbidities, such as diabetes, sleep apnea, hypertension, or Pickwickian syndrome. The American Society for Bariatric Surgery estimates that over 140,000 procedures were performed in 2004—up from 16,000 surgeries in 1993[1]—and that this number will continue to steadily rise.

WLS, also called bariatric surgery, requires lifelong management on the part of the patient and a skilled multidisciplinary medical team. Although surgery can produce excellent results of 50-[2] to over 80-percent[3] excess weight loss long-term and resolution of many comorbidities,[4] patients develop new risks as a direct result of the procedures.

Nutritional deficiencies are a clear danger after all types of WLS. While the risk varies with the procedure, none is immune. The ultimate goal of WLS is to create a greater opportunity for health and longevity. As powerful tools for the promotion of weight loss, these procedures increase patients' potential for better health. However, many patients and even physicians downplay the role of postoperative nutrition in long-term health and wellbeing. In the early months and years after a patient's WLS, when he or she is basking in the benefits of a thinner more mobile body and reversed comorbid conditions, it may be hard for that patient to think about the greatly increased risk for neurological impairment and bone loss that can result from poor nutrition. Despite the fact that nutritional deficiencies may sound like very small concerns when compared to hypertension, diabetes, sleep apnea, and the sheer stigma of morbid obesity, they are very real concerns for WLS patients. Unmonitored deficiencies can leave patients vulnerable to both acute and chronic conditions with variable reversibility and, in some cases, permanent physical damage.

Health professionals addressing the nutritional care of WLS patients are often asked to understand very complex nutritional science—potentially far beyond what they are taught in their formal education. Very few healthcare professionals have been taught to understand the therapeutic use of dietary supplements, which is a mainstay for postoperative WLS care. Additionally, nutritional diagnosis is not consistent across bariatric programs. Physicians may test only a small, select number of nutrients, which allows them to miss potentially serious problems. Finally, there is often confusion about how nutrient status should be evaluated and what constitutes the best testing methods for WLS patients.

The intent of this book is to focus on three key areas: Diagnosis, prevention, and intervention. Ideally, an emphasis on the first two areas can help minimize the need for the latter. One underlying theme of this book will be management, including timing and frequency of labs and follow-up, and strategies for promotion of adherence in nutritional programs.

If we step back from bariatric surgery for a moment and look merely at the available tools for promoting health and longevity in the general population, fitness and nutrition are very high on the list. Each cell of the human body operates on a complex set of chemical reactions that are dependent on nutritional cofactors. Of these cofactors, those that are deemed essential— including select proteins, fats, carbohydrates, vitamins, and minerals—are a daily requirement for maintaining normal cellular health and physiology. While we can survive without some or all of these on a very limited basis, deprivation over time creates both frank pathology and disease risk.

The concept of preventive medicine, especially preventive nutrition, is not new to medicine, but has barely begun to gain serious attention. For decades, the general paradigm of medicine that has been taught is that food can unquestionably provide adequate nutrition to meet individual health needs. Science, on the other hand, paints a different picture. The United States Department of Agriculture (USDA) has kept track of US micro- and macronutrient intake since 1909. They publish summaries of this information approximately every 10 years, much of which has been used to create programs, such as Dietary Guidelines for Americans, the Food Pyramid, and recommendations on food fortification. These documents contain valuable information about the nutritional content of the US food supply and the nutritional status of consumers (namely the US population). Some of the findings of the most recently published USDA survey from 1996 include the following:

- Over 70 percent of men and women failed to get even two-thirds of the recommended dietary allowance (RDA) for one or more nutrients.
- Only three percent of the population eats the recommended number of servings from the four food groups on each of three days.
- Only 12 percent of the population consumes 100 percent of the RDA for all seven of the following nutrients: Protein, calcium, iron, vitamin A, thiamin, riboflavin, and vitamin C.
- Not a single person consumed 100 percent of the RDA for all 10 of the following nutrients: Vitamin B6, Vitamin B12, magnesium, protein, calcium, iron, vitamin A, thiamin, riboflavin, and vitamin C.

In 2001, in the *New England Journal of Medicine*, Willet and Stamfer reviewed current evidence pointing to low-grade micronutrient deficiency in the US and concluded the following: "Given the greater likelihood of benefit than harm, and considering the low cost, we conclude that a daily multivitamin...makes sense for most adults...Substantial data suggest that higher intakes of folic acid, vitamin B6, vitamin B12, and vitamin D will benefit many people, and a multivitamin will ensure an adequate intake of other vitamins for which the evidence of benefit is indirect."[5]

A year later, a similar sentiment was echoed in the *Journal of the American Medical Association*. Fairfield and Fletcher reviewed studies published between 1996 and 2002 that examined the connection between vitamin intake and disease. Additionally, they reviewed far-reaching data, such as the USDA studies, and concluded that everyone, regardless of age or health status, needs a daily multivitamin. The following summarizes their ultimate opinion: "Most people do not consume optimal levels of all vitamins by diet alone. Pending strong evidence of effectiveness from randomized trials, it appears prudent for all adults to take vitamin supplements."[6,7]

Thus, we know that as a rule, Americans do not meet their basic nutritional needs through diet. Outside of the generally "healthy" population, we have evidence that specific disease states create further nutritional challenges. Obesity is an excellent example of this. In WLS patients specifically, there is evidence supporting nutritional deficits. One 1993 study[8] published in *Obesity Surgery* found that 62 percent of preoperative female patients had vitamin D deficiency. A 2005 study found the same in 51 percent of patients, with a higher incidence in dark-skinned individuals.[9] A recent evaluation of 303 preoperative patients found a 15.5-percent prevalence of thiamine deficiency prior to surgery.[10] A 1988 report in the *Journal of the American Dietetic Association* found preoperative deficiencies of vitamins E, B6, and folate.[11]

If these types of deficiencies exist prior to WLS, the procedures only serve to increase the nutritional risk to the patient. Diminished food intake, coupled with malabsorption and altered food profiles establishes an environment where deficiencies become increasingly likely in the absence of a sound nutritional strategy.

## HOW TO USE THIS BOOK

Nutritional medicine is really a specialty unto itself, and few physicians today are properly prepared to manage complex cases such as those that may present in WLS patients. This book is intended to be a clinical guide for surgeons, primary care physicians, dietitians, and others caring for WLS patients. It is not meant to provide a course in nutritional biochemistry, but rather is intended to be a practical manual for prevention, diagnosis, and treatment of nutritional deficiencies. While some protocol is included, clinicians using this book ultimately should find themselves better equipped to make their own educated decisions regarding nutritional management of their WLS patients.

## MY PERSONAL HOPE

As a naturopathic doctor, I have devoted my career to helping people not only to correct their acute and chronic health issues with minimally invasive treatments, but also to promoting prevention through diet, lifestyle, and nutrition. The goal of naturopathic medicine is to employ therapies that support and promote the body's natural healing process leading to the highest state of wellness. Naturopathic doctors also adhere to a set of philosophical guidelines, one of which is *tolle causum*, which means remove the cause. This principle states that major obstacles to health must be removed before health can be restored. I believe that WLS patients should be given every occasion to reach that highest state, and that surgery, by removing the obstacle of obesity and its comorbidities, is the first step.

WLS is about nothing if it is not about creating an opportunity for health. In their position paper titled *Rationale for the Surgical Treatment of Morbid Obesity*, the American Society for Bariatric Surgery correctly argues that, "...the option of surgical treatment [of obesity] is a rational one supported by the time-honored principle that diseases that harm call for therapeutic intervention that, while vigorous, is less harmful than the disease being treated."[12]

It should follow that all reasonable measures ought to be taken to assure that possible consequences of the procedures themselves do not cause patients to experience preventable new health problems. In other words, we must strive to reduce long-term harm to the patients being treated. Further, it might be possible to imagine a strategy where the goal goes beyond prevention of nutrient deficiency and toward health promotion. Following massive weight loss and reversal of serious comorbidities, WLS patients are poised to experience not only thinner bodies, but truly better health. Patients now have the opportunity to benefit, as many did not before, from the health effects of dietary modification, exercise, and nutritional supplementation. Extending the vision to one of long-term health and vitality also gives patients a positive goal for which to reach—one that moves them further from illness and closer to physical, mental, and emotional wellbeing. Do no harm, remove the obstacles to health, and give patients the tools to achieve what may otherwise have been impossible.

I hope this book can guide you to provide the best possible clinical care for the patients you treat.

In health,
*Jacqueline Jacques, ND*

# REFERENCES

1.  Blackburn G. Solutions in weight control: Lessons from gastric surgery. *Am J Clin Nutr* 2005;82(1):248S–52S.
2.  Spivak H, Hewitt M, Onn A, Half E. Weight loss and improvement of obesity-related illness in 500 US patients following laparoscopic adjustable gastric banding procedure. *Am J Surg* 2005;189(1):27–32.
3.  Burhop J, Chiang MC, Engstrand D, O'Driscoll M. Laparoscopic bariatric surgery can be performed safely in the community hospital setting. *WMJ* 2005;104(5):48–53.
4.  Buchwald H, Avidor Y, Braunwald E, et al. Bariatric surgery: A systematic review and meta-analysis. *JAMA* 2004;292(14):1724–37. Erratum in: *JAMA* 2005;293(14):1728.
5.  Willett WC, Stampfer, MJ. What vitamins should I be taking, Doctor? *NEJM* 2001;345:1819–24.
6.  Fairfield KM, Fletcher RH. Vitamins for chronic disease prevention in adults: Scientific review. *JAMA* 2002;287:3116–26.
7.  Fletcher RH Fairfield KM. Vitamins for chronic disease prevention in adults: Clinical applications. *JAMA* 2002;287:3127–9.
8.  Buffington C, Walker B, Cowan GS Jr, Scruggs D. Vitamin D deficiency in the morbidly obese. *Obes Surg* 1993;3(4):421–4.
9.  Carlin AM, et al. Prevalence of vitamin D deficiency among morbidly obese patients seeking gastric bypass surgery. *Surgery for Obesity and Related Diseases* 2005;1(3):243–4.
10. Antozzi P, et al. Thiamine deficiency in an obese population undergoing laparoscopic bariatric surgery. *Surgery for Obesity and Related Diseases* 2005;(3):264–65.
11. Boylan LM, Sugerman HJ, Driskell JA. Vitamin E, vitamin B6, vitamin B12, and folate status of gastric bypass surgery patients. *J Am Diet Assoc* 1988;88(5):579–85.
12. American Society of Bariatric Surgery. Rationale for the Surgical Treatment of Morbid Obesity. Available at: http://www.asbs.org/html/patients/rationale.html. Accessd date: 11/4/05.

# PART 1: Preoperative Nutrition

The time leading up to weight loss surgery (WLS) is a time of great opportunity. While patients are gathering information, undergoing needed medical exams, awaiting insurance approvals, and generally preparing for surgery, there are several areas where nutrition can play a valuable role.

The chapters in this section will focus on two areas: General nutritional preparation for surgery and nutrition for management of fatty liver—including preoperative weight loss. The goal generally is to have patients be prepared physically as well as psychologically for WLS.

## GENERAL PREOPERATIVE NUTRITION

There is a common perception that those who are overweight are eating more and are thus not likely to have nutritional deficiencies. When we actually look at nutrition in morbidly obese patients, however, we do not find this to be the case. Obesity creates nutritional demands on the human body that are over and beyond the normal requirements on which the dietary reference intakes (DRIs) are based. Some of this appears to be due to obesity-related comorbidities, such as diabetes, but other nutritional demands may be due to excess adipose tissue or reasons not yet understood. Additionally, it is important to recall our discussion from the Introduction that most Americans do not obtain adequate nutrition from diet alone. Add to this the further demands obesity places on the body, and the stage is set for distinct deficiencies to develop.

# CHAPTER 1

# Nutritional Deficiency in Obesity

O besity is the second most common preventable cause of death in the US, killing 10 times more people than motor vehicle accidents do[1] and approaching the number of deaths caused by cancer. Despite this, we still have a lot to learn about the condition itself. Textbooks on nutrition have historically utilized the term *over-nutrition* when referring to the condition of obesity. Although this term technically refers to weight gain that occurs due to an imbalance between caloric intake and energy expenditure, the term suggests that the overweight individual is better nourished than the average person.

In reality, we have limited knowledge of the true nutritional status of obese individuals. As cited in the introduction to this book, Americans generally favor calorie-dense, nutrient-poor diets that supply less than the recommended daily allowance (RDA) of many vitamins and minerals. We have growing reason to believe that obesity and some of its common comorbid conditions like diabetes create greater nutritional demands on the body, perhaps contributing to deficiency. Thus, obese individuals may have nutritional requirements that are over and above the normals on which the DRIs (Dietary Reference Intakes[2]) are based. Limited studies that have looked at overall nutritional status in obese populations have demonstrated that this is likely to be true,[3] but more data is needed to determine what nutritional challenges are a direct result of obesity versus those that may correlate with other factors, such as age or economic status.

## WHY IS THIS IMPORTANT?

Good nutritional status is a marker for good health. When patients are preparing for a major surgical procedure, their nutritional status may have an impact on both short- and long-term outcomes. Good nutritional status is important for normal wound healing, immunity, and recovery times, and some of the specific nutrients that have been shown to be impaired in obesity are directly correlated with these outcomes.[4-8] Following bariatric surgery, the early weeks and months present patients with varying degrees of challenges in nutrient intake, which may be complicated by episodes of vomiting and dumping syndrome. Moreover, risk for nutrient deficiencies continues to increase over time in patients with malabsorptive procedures, such as gastric bypass. Increasing our understanding of preoperative nutrition may lead not only to better patient health and improved recovery, but also to predictive models of who may be at greatest risk for early onset of postoperative nutritional deficiencies. This kind of information could eventually help to answer questions about why some patients develop acute nutritional problems while others remain healthy for years. Finally, healthier patients with better outcomes are good for the entire weight loss surgery (WLS) community. The more that can be done to assure patient health, the more successful everyone is.

## DEFICIENCIES LINKED TO OBESITY

### Antioxidant Nutrients
Antioxidants are nutrients or chemicals that neutralize free radicals in the body. Free radicals are unstable molecules containing unstable oxygen or nitrogen species that can damage cell membranes, deoxyribonucleic acid (DNA), and other molecular structures. Damage from free radicals is linked to aging, cancer, heart disease and other health problems. Dietary antioxidants are critical for maintaining and replenishing the overall antioxidant capacity of the body. They include many essential nutrients like vitamins C, A, E, selenium, and zinc, as well as phytochemicals like carotenoids, anthyocyanins, flavonoids, and catechins.

As scientists have begun to explore the links between obesity, cardiovascular disease, and metabolic syndrome, antioxidants have been studied as a possible link in the pathophysiological chain. When antioxidant status is low in the human body, this creates a condition known as oxidative stress. There is an established inverse relationship between oxidative stress and cardiovascular diseases, including angina,[9] atherosclerosis,[10] and coronary artery disease.[11] Low antioxidant status is also directly linked to oxidation of low-density lipoprotein (LDL) cholesterol, which is thought to be a necessary step in the development of atherosclerotic plaques.

Metabolic syndrome is a condition defined by a cluster of symptoms, including abdominal obesity, hypertension, insulin resistance, dyslipidemia, inflammation, and increased thrombic tendencies. While the definition includes the constellation of problems, obesity is thought to be a major factor in the development of the condition. Insulin-resistant individuals often have an increase in advanced glycation end-products (AGEs). AGEs act as free radicals, thus further stressing the endogenous antioxidant system. This, in turn, may create an even greater conditional need for antioxidants in these individuals.

Oxidative stress is generally more prevalent in obesity for these reasons and others that are not fully understood. It is likely that the cause for low antioxidant oxidant status is multifold, including additional causes, such as increased demand (due to increased free radical activity), fat sequestering of key antioxidant nutrients (discussed below), and possibly low intake.

## Vitamin E

Vitamin E is considered to be the most important fat-soluble antioxidant in humans. It plays a vital role in protecting cell membranes, acting as the chain-breaking antioxidant in the cascade of free-radical destruction of the cellular lipid bilayer. Additionally, it protects LDL from oxidation, influences cell-signaling, modulates inflammation, decreases platelet adhesiveness, and promotes vasodilation.

Numerous studies have confirmed low plasma vitamin E status in obesity.[12-14] It is believed that, similar to vitamin D deficiency in obesity, this may occur due to fat-soluble nutrients sequestering in adipose tissue, removing them from circulation, and resulting in functionally lowered status.[15]

## Carotenoids

Carotenoids are a collection of red, orange, and yellow-pigmented compounds found throughout the human diet. Some, like beta-carotene, are vitamin A precursors. Approximately 26 to 34 percent of dietary vitamin A comes from sources like beta-carotene.[16] Other carotenoids, such as lutein, lycopene, and zeaxanthin, do not convert to vitamin A, but act as significant antioxidants in their own right. In addition to acting as a source of vitamin A, carotenoids help to protect LDL from oxidation, filter ultraviolet light in the retina, support immune health, and facilitate intracellular communication.

Most of the same studies that have examined vitamin E status have also measured carotenoids and vitamin A (retinol). Universally, carotenoids are found to be low in a similar pattern to vitamin E. Interestingly, levels of retinol appear to be normal in obesity. If part of the genesis of low E and carotenoids is storage in adipose tissue, why would deficiency of retinol—also a fat-soluble antioxidant—not be present? This is likely due to the differences in absorption, transport, and storage of the nutrient forms. Retinol is largely stored in the liver[17] while carotenoids are stored in adipocytes.[18] It is also interesting to note that conversion of carotenoids to retinol is impaired in both hypothyroidism and diabetes, conditions common in obesity. Therefore, it maybe possible that these conditions further serve to keep body stores of carotenoids sequestered in adipose tissue by not allowing for efficient conversion to retinol in affected individuals.

## Vitamin C

Vitamin C is a key nutritional antioxidant protecting cell membranes, DNA, proteins, and carbohydrates from free radical damage. It also acts to regenerate other antioxidants (e.g., vitamin E), which become potent free radicals themselves after performing their antioxidant function. Additionally, vitamin C is required for the structural integrity of collagen, bone, and blood vessels. It is used in the synthesis of both norepinepherine and carnitine, helps to transport fatty acids into the cellular mitochondria, and assists with the metabolism of cholesterol to bile acids.

A couple of modest studies have confirmed low vitamin C levels in obesity.[19,20] A mechanism for this has not been proposed, but increased oxidative stress, as discussed previously, may be the primary axis.

## Zinc

Zinc is an essential trace mineral that is a structural component of over 100 enzymes in the human body. Some of these, like copper-zinc superoxide dismutase (CuZn-SOD), are important antioxidants. Zinc is also believed to act as an antioxidant in cell membranes, especially in the nervous system. When zinc levels are low, cell membranes are more susceptible to free radical damage.[21]

One 2002 study examined oxidative stress zinc status in obese male patients and found a positive correlation between obesity, increased oxidative stress, and impaired CuZn-SOD activity in conjunction with low cellular zinc levels. Outside of increased antioxidant demand due to oxidative stress, other mechanisms for deficiency were not proposed. Mild zinc deficiency has been verified in diabetes, which may be a contributing cause.[22]

## Homocysteine, B12, and Folate

Homocysteine is a byproduct of methionine metabolism that is an independent risk factor for vascular disease, stroke, heart attack, and birth defects. Elevations are also associated with dementia, some forms of inflammatory arthritis, depression, and osteoporosis. Homocysteine is normally metabolized to S-adenosylmethionine (SAMe) through the process of methylation using vitamins B12 and folate as methyl donors. This can also be accomplished with the methyl donor betaine (trimethylglycine). An alternate pathway utilizes vitamin B6 and ultimately results in the creation of cysteine.

Because of the strong association with cardiovascular disease, studies have attempted to explore a causative relationship between low B-vitamins, elevated homocysteine, obesity, and metabolic syndrome. To date, there is no strong evidence that obesity alone produces elevated homocysteine. There is, however, evidence of both elevated homocysteine[24] and low folate[25,26] in obese patients with metabolic syndrome.

### Thiamine

Thiamine, also known as vitamin B1, is a nutrient of growing concern after WLS.[27] It is interesting, therefore, that a 2005 study conducted at the Cleveland Clinic Florida demonstrated a 15.5-percent deficiency rate in morbidly obese patients presenting for WLS. Reasons for this deficiency may be multifold. Poor dietary intake cannot be ruled out as a partial cause.[28,29] Alcohol intake as well as long-term use of aminoglycosides, digoxin, fluoroquinolones, loop diuretics, phenytoin, penicillin, sulfonamides, tetracycline, and trimethoprim[30] are all risks for impaired thiamine status. Moreover, impaired glucose status and consumption of a diet high in carbohydrates are significant risk factors. Thiamine is a critical nutrient for the conversion of blood sugar into cellular energy. Increased blood sugars or excess intake can create a functional shortage in thiamine due to increased demand.

### Vitamin D

Vitamin D is an important nutrient for maintaining body calcium balance. It also plays a role in cell differentiation and communication, immunity, insulin secretion, and regulation of blood pressure. Obesity is an established risk factor for vitamin D deficiency.[31] Vitamin D deficiency has been directly demonstrated in two studies of preoperative WLS patients. One 1993 study published in *Obesity Surgery*[32] found that 62 percent of preoperative female patients had vitamin D deficiency. A 2005 study found a preoperative deficiency in 51 percent of patients, with a higher incidence in dark-skinned individuals.[33] The likely cause of this deficiency in obesity is believed to be the sequestering of vitamin D (both that which is ingested in the diet and quantities synthesized in the skin) in body fat stores.[34]

## RECOMMENDATIONS

Detailed nutritional testing prior to WLS may be hard to justify outside of facilities engaged in the collection of clinical data for research. Comprehensive evaluations of this kind are costly. It does appear, however, that we have enough early data to advise nutritional counseling prior to WLS. This is likely to have multiple benefits for both patient and clinician.

Patients typically have a wait time of several months (or longer) between making a decision to have bariatric surgery and the procedure itself. During this time insurance approvals are sought, necessary tests (e.g., cardiac risk assessments and psychological evaluations) are performed, and patients are often provided with education to prepare them for what lies ahead. This time can also be used to help prepare patients for surgery. Some programs require attendance of support groups, initiation of an exercise regimen, or weight loss. Given the probability that some level of nutritional impairment is likely to be present in preoperative patients, this time could also be used to help patients build nutrient stores.

In the absence of significant diagnostic testing, advising patients to take a daily multivitamin supplement is probably the most common sense recommendation. There are few studies that assess the health outcomes of daily multivitamin use outside of discrete populations (pregnant women, HIV infected individuals, malnourished children, etc.); however, a 2003 study published in the *Annals of Internal Medicine* highlights the potential for this intervention. In the study, 154 adults, ages 40 to 64, were stratified into treatment (a daily multivitamin) or no-treatment groups. In each group, approximately 70 percent were overweight or obese, and 30 percent had type 2 diabetes. After 12 months, the most significant findings in the study demonstrated significantly improved immunity among the vitamin group (73% vs. 43%). When further analyzed, the data showed that the patients with diabetes accounted for virtually 100 percent of this effect. A full 93 percent of patients with diabetes in the control group reported infections compared to 17 percent of patients without diabetes in the control group. Considering the high association between obesity, insulin resistance, and type 2 diabetes, this study is the closest we have to a preoperative bariatric surgery population. In their 2002 review of nutrition intake in US adults, Fairfield and Fletcher concluded the following:

"Most people do not consume optimal levels of all vitamins by diet alone. Pending strong evidence of effectiveness from randomized trials, it appears prudent for all adults to take vitamin supplements."[35,36]

Given the safety and economy of the intervention, coupled with the potential benefits to patients, vitamin supplementation is certainly something clinicians should consider.

The further question of whether patients should be given more thorough evaluations or intensive supplemental regimens cannot really be answered at this time. Clearly, when there is evidence of deficiency in an individual patient, such as a frank anemia, measures should be taken to correct the problem prior to surgery, and these patients should be monitored more closely for recurrence after surgery. It is also worth noting that there is a small but growing trend of treating preoperative vitamin D deficiency. It is not yet known whether this will result in better postoperative status, but hopefully further study will provide this information.

Unless another condition would warrant otherwise, a general multivitamin providing the following should be adequate:

1.   100 to 200 percent of the daily value (DV) for thiamin, riboflavin, folic acid, niacin, pantothenic acid, vitamin B6, vitamin B12, biotin, chromium, copper, iodine, manganese, molybdenum, and zinc. Those with iodine sensitivity should seek iodine-free vitamins.
2.   2500 to 5000IU of vitamin A. It is best if no more than half comes from retinol.
3.   Vitamin C in the range of 60 to 500mg.
4.   Vitamin D in the range of 400 to 600IU.
5.   Vitamin E in the range of 30 to 200IU. If a patient is taking blood thinners, the lower end of this range may be more appropriate. While some surgeons will feel more comfortable advising discontinuation of vitamin E-containing products 1 to 4 weeks prior to surgery, they should be made aware that this is only known to be a problem at levels well above 800IU in the absence of vitamin K deficiency. In the absence of vitamin K deficiency, the Institute of Medicine sets the level of 1500IU as the highest dose unlikely to result in bleeding.
6.   Vitamin K at approximately the DV of 80mcg. This should be avoided, however, in those taking anticoagulants.
7.   Iron at the level of the RDA (18mg) for menstruating women. Men and menopausal women do not need iron preoperatively.

8.   Selenium in the range of 70 to 200mcg.
9.   Calcium and magnesium levels in a multivitamin almost never come close to the DV because they are very large nutrients and take up a lot of space. Some should be present. It would not be harmful for patients to take additional calcium and magnesium up to the level of the DV at the discretion of the healthcare practitioner.
10.  Chloride, phosphorus, and potassium are sometimes present, but are so plentiful in the human diet that they are not usually required.
11.  Other nutrients may include boron, vanadium, silicon, tin, nickel, choline, or inositol, which are fine in modest amounts.

# REFERENCES

1.   Mokdad AH, Marks JS, Stroup DF, et al. Actual causes of death in the United States, 2000. *JAMA* 2004;291:1238–45.
2.   The DRIs are actually a set of four reference values: Estimated Average Requirements (EAR), Recommended Dietary Allowances (RDA), Adequate Intakes (AI), and Tolerable Upper Intake Levels, (UL), which have replaced the 1989 Recommended Dietary Allowances (RDAs).
3.   Ledikwe JH, Smiciklas-Wright H, Mitchell DC, et al. Nutritional risk assessment and obesity in rural older adults: A sex difference. *Am J Clin Nutr* 2003;77(3):551–8.
4.   Swartz-Basile DA, Rubin DC, Levin MS. Vitamin A status modulates intestinal adaptation after partial small bowel resection. *J Parenter Enteral Nutr* 2000;24:81–8.
5.   Thomas DR. Specific nutritional factors in wound healing. *Adv Wound Care* 1997;10:40–3 [review].
6.   Senapati A, Slavin BM, Thompson RPH. Zinc depletion and complications of surgery. *Clin Nutr* 1990;9:341–6.
7.   Zunic J, Stavljenic-Rukavina A, Granic P, et al. Changes in vitamin E concentration after surgery and anesthesia. *Coll Antropol* 1997;21:327–34.
8.   Thomas DR. Specific nutritional factors in wound healing. *Adv Wound Care* 1997;10:40–3 [review].
9.   Riemersma RA, Wood DA, Macintyre CCH, et al. Risk of angina pectoris and plasma concentrations of vitamins A, C, and E, and carotene. *Lancet* 1991;337:1–5.
10.  Diaz MN, Frei B, Vita JA, Keaney JF. Antioxidants and atherosclerotic heart disease. *N Engl J Med* 1997;337:408–15.
11.  Stampfer MJ, Hennekens CH, Manson JE, et al. Vitamin E consumption and the risk of coronary disease in women. *N Engl J Med* 1993;328:1444–8.
12.  Reitman A, Friedrich I, Ben-Amotz A, Levy Y. Low plasma antioxidants and normal plasma B vitamins and homocysteine in patients with severe obesity. *Isr Med Assoc J* 2002;4(8):590–3.
13.  Morinobu T, Murata T, Takaya R, Tamai H. Nutritional status of beta-carotene, alpha-tocopherol and retinol in obese children. *Int J Vitam Nutr Res* 2002;72(3):119–23.
14.  Ohrvall M, Tengblad S, Vessby B. Lower tocopherol serum levels in subjects with abdominal adiposity. *J Intern Med* 1993;234:53–60.
15.  Reitman A, Friedrich I, Ben-Amotz A, Levy Y. Low plasma antioxidants and normal plasma B vitamins and homocysteine in patients with severe obesity. *Isr Med Assoc J* 2002;4(8):590–3.
16.  Institute of Medicine. Food and Nutrition Board. Dietary Reference Intakes for Vitamin A, Vitamin K, Arsenic, Boron, Chromium, Copper, Iodine, Iron, Manganese, Molybdenum, Nickel, Silicon, Vanadium, and Zinc. Washington, DC: National Academy Press, 2001.
17.  Ross AC. Vitamin A. In: Shils M, Olson J, Shike M, Ross AC (eds). *Modern Nutrition in Health and Disease, Ninth Edition.* Shils M, Olson J, Shike M, Ross AC (eds). Baltimore, MD: Williams & Wilkins, 1999:305–13.
18.  Bucci LR. Dietary supplements as ergogenic aids. In: Wolinksy I (ed). *Nutrition in Exercise and Sport, Third Edition.* New York: CRC Press, 1998:328–9.
19.  Harnroongroj T, Jintaridhi P, Vudhivai N, et al. B vitamins, vitamin C, and hematological measurements in overweight and obese Thais in Bangkok. *Med Assoc Thai* 2002;85(1):17–25.
20.  de Burgos AM, Wartanowicz M, Ziemlanowski S. Blood vitamin and lipid levels in overweight and obese women. *Eur J Clin Nutr* 1992;46:803–8.
21.  O'Dell BL. Role of zinc in plasma membrane function. *J Nutr* 2000;130(5S Suppl):1432S–6S.
22.  Chausmer AB. Zinc, insulin, and diabetes. *J Am Coll Nutr* 1998;17(2):109–15.
23.  Reitman A, Friedrich I, Ben-Amotz A, Levy Y. Low plasma antioxidants and normal plasma B vitamins and homocysteine in patients with severe obesity. *Isr Med Assoc J* 2002;4(8):590–3.
24.  Harnroongroj T, Jintaridhi P, Vudhivai N, et al. B vitamins, vitamin C, and hematological measurements in overweight and obese Thais in Bangkok. *Med Assoc Thai* 2002;85(1):17–25.
25.  Hirsch S, Poniachick J, Avendano M, et al. Serum folate and homocysteine levels in obese females with non-alcoholic fatty liver. *Nutrition* 2005;21(2):137–41.
26.  Ledikwe JH, Smiciklas-Wright H, Mitchell DC, et al. Nutritional risk assessment and obesity in rural older adults: A sex

difference. *Am J Clin Nutr* 2003;77(3):551–8.

27.   Antozzi P. Thiamine deficiency in an obese population undergoing laparoscopic bariatric surgery. *Surg Obes Rel Dis* 2005;1(3):264–5.

28.   Lonsdale D, Schamberger RJ. Red cell transketolase as indicator of nutritional deficiency. *Am J Clin Nutr* 1980;33:205–11.

29.   Chen MF, Chen LT, Gold M, Boyce HW Jr. Plasma and erythrocyte thiamin concentration in geriatric outpatients. *J Am Coll Nutr* 1996:15:231–6.

30.   Pelton R, LaValle JB, Hawkins E, Krinsky DL (eds). *Drug-Induced Nutrient Depletion Handbook.* Hudson, OH: Lexi-Comp, 1999:258.

31.   Arunabh S, Pollack S, Yeh J, Aloia JF. Body fat content and 25-hydroxyvitamin D levels in healthy women. *J Clin Endocrinol Metab* 2003;88(1):157–61.

32.   Buffington C, Walker B, Cowan GS Jr, Scruggs D. Vitamin D deficiency in the morbidly obese. *Obes Surg* 1993;3(4):421–4.

33.   Carlin AM. Prevalence of vitamin D deficiency among morbidly obese patients seeking gastric bypass surgery. *Surg ObesRel Dis* 2005;1(3):243–4.

34.   Arunabh S, Pollack S, Yeh J, Aloia JF. Body fat content and 25-hydroxyvitamin D levels in healthy women. *J Clin Endocrinol Metab* 2003;88(1):157–61.

35.   Fairfield KM, Fletcher RH. Vitamins for chronic disease prevention in adults: Scientific review. *JAMA* 2002;287:3116–26.

36.   Fletcher RH, Fairfield KM. Vitamins for chronic disease prevention in adults: Clinical applications. *JAMA* 2002;287:3127–9.

37.   Food and Nutrition Board, Institute of Medicine. Vitamin E. Dietary reference intakes for vitamin C, vitamin E, selenium, and carotenoids. Washington DC: National Academy Press, 2000:186–283.

# CHAPTER 2

# Nutrition in the Management of Non-alcoholic Fatty Liver

Non-alcoholic fatty liver disease (NAFLD), which includes non-alcoholic steatohepatitis (NASH), is common in patients qualifying for weight loss surgery (WLS). Risk factors for NAFLD include obesity, diabetes, and insulin resistance. Of these, obesity is considered to be the greatest single risk factor. Incidence of NAFLD in patients with obesity or type 2 diabetes can be as high as 90 percent.[1] It is estimated that between 50 and 60 percent of preoperative bariatric surgery patients meet the diagnostic criteria for NASH.[2]

The enlargement of the liver due to fatty infiltration and, in the case of NASH, inflammation, can significantly interfere with the surgical field in WLS procedures. Obscuring of the surgical field, especially portions of the stomach, can prolong surgical times, increasing risk to the patient. Inability to retract the liver in a laparoscopic procedure is cited as the single most common cause for conversion to an open procedure, accounting for roughly half of such conversions,[3] according to some reports.

## DIAGNOSIS

Liver biopsy and histology are currently the only accurate ways to diagnose NAFLD. Precise, noninvasive screening for NAFLD and NASH in preoperative patients still has not been demonstrated. Laboratory studies have not proven to be accurate predictors. Amonitransferases (aspartate aminotransferase [AST] or alanine aminotransferase [ALT]) may be elevated, but can also be normal. The same is true for alkaline phosphatase, hyperlipidemia, and serum triglycerides. Elevated fasting insulin may be a more sensitive marker, especially if other evidence of insulin resistance exists (elevated triglycerides, hypertension, and central obesity). Some studies have shown elevated serum ferritin or serum iron to be a relatively common finding in NASH. If this is present, patients should likely undergo additional evaluation to rule out hemochromatosis.

Imaging studies can contribute to a diagnosis of NAFLD, but may be challenging or even impossible in larger patients. Ultrasound, computed tomography (CT), and contrast magnetic resonance imaging (MRI) can all identify fatty liver to some degree. The accuracy of ultrasound is significantly affected by the presence of fatty tissue.[4] Both CT and MRI are limited by patient weight and girth. CT weight limits are in the range of 425 to 450 pounds with a limit of 87 inches in body circumference; MRIs have a general weight range of 300 to 450 pounds and a body circumference limit of 74 inches. While open MRIs may accommodate larger patients, the image is weaker and less accurate for this diagnosis.

Because of the diagnostic challenges, coupled with high rate of occurrence, presumed diagnosis is not uncommon in programs wishing to implement precautionary interventions, such as preoperative weight loss. Some programs limit these interventions to patients with higher body mass index (BMI), greater waist circumference, or those meeting the diagnostic criteria for metabolic syndrome. A study conducted by Dixon, et al.,[5] in preoperative WLS patients found insulin resistance and hypertension—the diagnostic features of metabolic syndrome—to have a high association with more advanced cases of NASH in the morbidly obese. As patients who are both obese and meet the diagnostic criteria for metabolic syndrome are statistically most likely to have fatty liver, this may be the easiest, most cost-effective screen currently available.

## THERAPEUTICS

According to the American Association for the Study of Liver Disease clinical practice guidelines, "There are no published controlled trials of treatment modalities for NAFLD. It is, therefore, not possible to make any statements on relative risk of improvement with any modality. In the absence of treatment modalities of proven efficacy, therapy is directed toward correction of the risk factors for NASH (i.e., insulin resistance, decreasing delivery of fatty acids to the liver, and decreasing use of drugs with potentially hepatotoxic effects)."

It is important to keep in mind that in relation to WLS the intent of treating NAFLD is not for lifelong management of the condition itself but rather is to reduce liver volume such that the surgery itself is easier for the surgeon, with a lower risk of complications for the patient. The fact is that most emerging data on NAFLD in obesity points to surgery itself an important option (if not the best option) for treatment of this condition.

## Weight Reduction

Weight loss is the most widely accepted therapy for NAFLD, and many surgical programs are beginning to recognize that even small losses of body weight can eliminate close to 100 percent of liver concerns that relate to surgery. While some studies have linked rapid weight reduction to increased liver inflammation, this risk appears to be low in short-term, medically monitored conditions such as would be used in preoperative patients.[6] In their report titled "Effects of Weight Loss Surgeries on Liver Disease,"[7] Blackburn and Mun recommend that, "All WLS patients should be encouraged to lose weight prior to surgery. Those with a BMI of >50kg/m$^2$ or such comorbidities as sleep apnea, type 2 diabetes, glucose intolerance, and hypertension should attempt to lose 5 to 10 percent of their initial weight."

There is currently no agreement on the degree, duration, or method of weight loss for reduction of NAFLD in preoperative patients. A single study examined the effects of an eight-percent weight loss in obese women with insulin resistance and high liver fat content compared to an equally obese control group. Weight was lost on a low calorie (600–800Kcal/day) formula diet, over a 2- to 3-month period. The group of women with high liver fat and insulin resistance demonstrated preferential loss of liver fat stores over loss of peripheral fat stores.[8] In those who do present with elevated liver enzymes, weight loss of 10 percent of total body weight has both normalized enzymes levels and reversed liver enlargement.[9] A 10-percent weight loss is also recommended by the National Heart, Lung, and Blood Institute-National Institute of Diabetes and Digestive Kidney Diseases (NHLBI-NIDDK).

This study and others have used low calorie formula diets with success. There is currently a substantial selection of formula diets available to clinicians. There is no substantial evidence that any one program would be of greater value for this purpose than any other. Factors such as cost to the patient (insurance does not usually cover the cost of product) and ease of use should be taken into account. It is advisable to seek products that are designed for medical use as meal replacements, as these products must meet specified formula requirements for nutritional content. Alternately, calorie-restricted food programs can be attempted, but there is less research to support their efficacy in the treatment of NAFLD.

Because evidence indicates that losing weight too rapidly may increase liver inflammation and, in rare cases, precipitate liver failure, the NHLBI-NIDDK advises that weight loss not exceed 3.5 pounds per week. Morbidly obese patients often lose more rapidly than this in the early weeks of a low or very low calorie diet. Serological tests, including liver function tests, do not appear to be accurate for the assessment of liver inflammation in these patients.[10] Fortunately, the studies that have assessed these changes through biopsy generally report the majority of cases to show only slight worsening of inflammation or fibrosis, while still demonstrating significant hepatic fat loss.[11] With continued weight loss, which will occur after WLS, inflammation and fibrosis almost universally improve. Generally, clinicians should be aware of the risk and may consider increased frequency of visits with patients reporting more rapid weight loss. As more bariatric surgeons now routinely collect liver biopsies, we may eventually be able to compare the liver histology of patients who have undergone preoperative weight loss with those who have not. This data, when available, will allow us to understand the real risk (if present) to WLS patients.

## Pharmacologic Therapies

Drugs that improve insulin resistance, such as biguanides (metformin) and thiazolidinediones (rosiglitazone and pioglitazone), have drawn interest for the treatment of NAFLD, as have some lipid-lowering agents and ursodeoxycholic acid (UDCA). Metformin has been shown to lower liver enzyme levels in patients with NAFLD at a dose of 500mg three times daily.[12] Among early trials of thiazolidinediones, troglitazone had shown some promise before being removed from the market for, interestingly, liver toxicity. Similarly, rosiglitazone[13] and pioglitazone[14] have demonstrated improvement in small pilot studies. All of these agents likely deserve further study.

The lipid-lowering agent atorvastatin has been evaluated in NAFLD treatment, and early data indicates it may be of benefit for patients who have significant hypercholesterolemia.[15,16] Gemfibrozil has been shown to lower liver enzymes in NASH patients.[17] Potentially more promising is ursodeoxycholic acid (UDCA). A naturally occurring bile acid, UDCA was evaluated in a controlled trial in NASH patients and was associated with lowering of liver enzymes and decreased liver fat content.[18] However, a later randomized trial showed no significant benefit over placebo.[19]

## Supportive Nutrition

The use of natural therapeutics in the management of NAFLD and NASH has largely focused on hepatoprotective agents. Use of substances that protect the liver and reduce liver inflammation may make sense in conjunction with weight loss, since increased liver inflammation is a known risk. It is believed that the increase in liver inflammation and fibrosis seen with more accelerated weight loss is likely due to rapid mobilization of free fatty acids. These fatty acids are metabolized through mitochondrial β–oxidation, which produces hydrogen peroxide and lipid peroxides—potent free-radicals. Individuals with NAFLD and NASH are already likely to have a higher degree of oxidative stress in the liver and higher levels of lipid peroxides. This additional, if only temporary, elevation in free fatty acid burden increases inflammation by placing further demands on an already stressed system.

### Vitamin E

As previously discussed in the section on nutrition and obesity, vitamin E is a potent fat-soluble antioxidant known to effectively combat lipid peroxidation. Since lipid peroxides are thought to be primary in the pathogenesis of liver injury in NASH, several clinical trials have sought to validate the use of vitamin E in this condition. In an open-label trial in a pediatric population, a dose of 400IU of vitamin E was initiated at the start of a three-month trial. Vitamin E was increased by an additional 400IU each month when transaminases levels remained elevated. Five of 11 participants demonstrated normalization of enzymes after one month; an additional four participants demonstrated normalization after two months; and all 11 participants had returned to normal by the end of the third month. No changes in liver size or fatty infiltration were seen on ultrasound, indicating that the effect of vitamin E therapy was to reduce inflammatory changes only.[20] A more recent study of 28 children had similar results with a dosage of 100 to 400IUs.[21] A second study evaluated the combination of vitamin E with a weight reduction diet in 22 obese adults.[22] Presence

| NATIONAL CHOLESTEROL EDUCATION PROGRAM ADULT TREATMENT PANEL (NCEP/ATP) III DEFINITION | WORLD HEALTH ORGANIZATION (WHO) DEFINITION |
|---|---|
| **Three or more of the following:** | **Diabetes, IGT, IFG, or insulin resistance, plus 2 or more of the following:** |
| *Waist circumference*<br>102cm (>40 in) in men<br>88cm (>35 in) in women | *Body mass index*<br>>30kg/m$^2$ and/or<br>*Waist-to-hip ratio*<br>>0.9 in men<br>>0.85 in women |
| *Triglycerides*<br>150mg/dL | *Triglycerides*<br>150mg/dL and/or |
| *HDL-C*<br><40mg/dL in men<br><50mg/dL in women | *HDL-C*<br><35mg/dL in men<br><39mg/dL in women |
| *Blood pressure*<br>130/85mmHg | *Blood pressure*<br>140/90mmHg |
| *FPG*<br>>100 mg/dL | *Microalbuminuria*<br>UAE [3]20mg/min or<br>*Albumin*<br>creatinine [3]30mg/g |

of NAFLD or NASH was determined by biopsy. After six months of weight loss, 300IU per day of vitamin E was added for 12 months. At the end of this time, repeat biopsies demonstrated significant improvement in both inflammation and fibrosis in 5 of 12 patients and decreased steatosis in an additional four. The inflammatory marker transforming growth factor-β1 (TGF-β1) was found to be unchanged with weight loss alone, but significantly reduced after vitamin E therapy.

*Vitamin E with C*

Several studies have sought to evaluate the combination of high-dose vitamin E and C in NASH with mixed results. Vitamin E and vitamin C are nutrient synergists. When vitamin E neutralizes a free radical and, in turn, generates the potent tocopherol radical, vitamin C is one of the antioxidants that can regenerate vitamin E to the non-radical state. A 2003 study placed 45 patients with NASH (diagnosed by biopsy) on a weight loss regimen together with 1000IU of vitamin E and

---

**PREOPERATIVE NUTRITIONAL SUPPORT FOR WEIGHT LOSS SURGERY PATIENTS**

**Basic Support**
- Daily multivitamin (see guidelines in Appendix A]
- Consider added calcium up to 1000 to 1500mg/day
- Additional specific nutrients if deficiencies are present

**Support for NAFLD**

- **Weight loss with formula diet (low or very low calorie) with goal of 5 to 10 percent weight loss**

- **Consider concurrent pharmacotherapy with:**
  *-Metformin*
  *-Atorvastatin*

- **Consider concurrent nutritional therapy with:**
  *-Vitamin E, 100–800IU d-alpha-tocopherol*
  *-Vitamin C, 1000mg*
  *-N-acetyl Cysteine, 1000—3000mg/day (in divided doses)*
  *-Betaine or SAMe—for betaine, 20 grams/day; for SAMe, consider 800—1200mg per day*
  *(the amounts studied in alcoholic liver disease).*

- **Strategies for patients with high triglycerides**
  *-Essential Fatty Acids—2 to 4 grams/day of omega-3 fatty acids from fish oil sources*
  *-Pantethine—600 to 900mg (given as 300mg BID to TID)*

- **Additional Possibilities**
  *-Milk Thistle, 600mg BID*
  *-Probiotics, no standard dosing as this depends on colony-forming units (CFUs) in the product being taken. Look for studied strains such as* Lactobacillus acidophilus, Lactobacillus casei, *or* Lactobacillus ruterii.

---

1000mg of vitamin C.[23] After six months, repeat histology demonstrated significant reduction in liver fibrosis, yet liver enzymes remained unchanged. Of two small additional trials, only one was able to reproduce similar results.[24] It is uncertain why the researchers chose to use such a high dose of vitamin E, given that the successful trials (cited previously) used much lower doses. The risk of excessive vitamin E is creation of very high levels of tocopherol radical, which may itself act as a free radical and inflammatory agent. Since the exact dose of vitamin C needed to recycle this amount of vitamin E cannot be accurately predicted, it may have been more logical to use a dose of vitamin E already known to produce desirable results in NASH. Hopefully, future studies will give greater consideration to antioxidant homeostasis.

*N-acetylcysteine (NAC)*

N-acetylcysteine is a sulfur-containing antioxidant and is the primary precursor to hepatic glutathione. NAC is a well established hepatoprotective agent and is best known in the medical world for its therapeutic use as an antidote to acetaminophen-induced liver toxicity. One small three-month trial of 1000mg per day of NAC showed markedly lowered transaminase levels in NASH patients.[25] NAC has also been shown to benefit insulin sensitivity at doses of 1.8 to 3 grams per day.[26] NAC is an extremely safe antioxidant with well understood pharmacokinetics. The LD-50 is greater than 6000mg/kg in rodent models, and no teratogenic evidence has been seen at doses as high as 2000mg/kg in animal fertility studies.[27] More studies of NAC in NAFLD should be considered.

### Betaine and SAMe

Betaine, also known as trimethylglycine, is a natural metabolite of choline. Betaine is known to act as a methyl donor and is able to raise levels of S-adenosylmethionine (SAMe). It is also one of the nutrients, along with B12, folate, and B6, that can recycle homocysteine back into methionine in the liver. High homocysteine is found commonly in patients with metabolic syndrome and is often found to be elevated in NASH.[28] Past studies have shown much promise for the use of SAMe in alcoholic liver disease.[29] One small trial in 10 patients with NASH followed both biopsies and liver enzymes in patients taking 20 grams per day of a betaine oral solution for one year. Significant reductions were seen in enzymes levels, as well as in fibrosis, inflammation, and fatty depositions in the liver.[30] Hypothetically, the use of SAMe itself might also prove effective. Other nutritional methyl donors, such as folate or vitamin B12, may hold potential, especially inpatients with high homocysteine.

## Other Possible Therapeutic Agents

### Pantethine

Pantethine is a natural derivative of pantothenic acid (vitamin B5). Pantethine is marketed in both Europe and Asia as a therapeutic agent for lowering cholesterol and triglycerides; in the United States it is considered to be a dietary supplement. Daily doses of 600 to 1200 milligrams have been demonstrated to effectively lower total cholesterol, low density lipoprotein (LDL) cholesterol, apolipoprotein B, and tryglicerides.[31,32] Some studies have also demonstrated elevated HDL.[33] Sixteen patients presenting with both NAFLD and elevated triglycerides were given 600mg of pantethine for six months.[34] Evaluation using abdominal CT scan showed complete resolution of fatty liver at the end of the study. Researchers found a corresponding increase in subcutaneous fat and hypothesized that fat mobilized from the liver and viscera was redistributed to subcutaneous deposits.

### Omega-3 Fatty Acids

The omega-3 fatty acids, eicosapentanoic acid (EPA) and docosahexanoic acid (DHA), from fish oil are proven to be helpful in the management of dyslipidemias, especially in high triglycerides.[35] Therapeutic doses for lowering triglycerides fall between 2 and 4 grams of fish oils per day.[36] In a trial that compared use of omega-3 fats to atorvastatin and orlistat in patients with NAFLD and hyperlipidemia, 23 patients were placed into the omega-3 arm. Patients were selected for this therapy if they presented with primary hypertriglyceridemia. For 24 weeks, participants took 5mL of an omega-3 oil containing 751mg of EPA and 527mg of DHA. After 24 weeks, all patients had reductions in triglycerides, cholesterol levels, and liver enzymes. Thirty-five percent of the omega-3 group reverted to normal findings on ultrasound (compared to 86% of patients receiving orlistat and 61% of those on atorvastatin). Given the overall health benefits of omega-3 fats and the short duration in which improvement was seen, this would appear to be a potentially useful intervention in appropriate patients.

*Probiotics*

Probiotics are beneficial microorganisms that reside in the digestive tract and are thought to play a role in digestive health and immunity. Probiotics have long been available as dietary supplements and can be obtained from cultured foods like yogurt. Common strains include *Bifidobacterium bifidum, Bifidobacterium longum, Lactobacillus acidophilus, Lactobacillus casei, Lactobacillus ruterii*, and *Saccharomyces boulardi*.

Interest in the use of probiotics to treat NAFLD has a historical connection to WLS and the now obsolete jejunoileal bypass (JIB) procedure. JIB fell from medical favor due to the high risk of developing complications, including diarrhea, night blindness, osteomalacia, protein-calorie malnutrition, and kidney stones. However, the worst complications, including inflammatory arthritis, dermatitis, malaise and serious liver pathology (ranging from steatosis to liver failure), were caused by overgrowth of toxin-producing bacteria in the gut.[37] It was realized that in some of these cases, liver damage could be reversed through the use of metronidazole to kill the abnormal flora.

Medically, the presence of these abnormal flora is referred to as small intestinal bacterial overgrowth (SIBO). Later animal models of SIBO produced hepatic lesions identical to those found both in JIB patients and in NASH.[38] It is now proposed that endotoxins produced by SIBO create liver inflammation and injury through the production of pro-inflammatory cytokines (namely TNF-$\alpha$) and the promotion of free radicals. A 2001 study in NASH patients confirmed that half of them had findings for SIBO compared to 22 percent of controls.[39] A study in a rodent model of NASH used probiotics or TNF-$\alpha$ antibodes and found improved liver histology and lower liver enzymes in both groups. It is believed that therapeutic use of beneficial probiotics can restore normal floral balance to the intestines, thereby eliminating toxin-producing species.

Currently the National Institutes of Health is funding a phase II clinical trial at Johns Hopkins University to evaluate the efficacy of probiotics in humans with NASH.

*Milk thistle*

The herbal medicine milk thistle is known by the botanical names *Silybum mariabum* (var. *albiflorum*). Medical herbalists use the term *Silymarin* to refer to both species. Most commercial products sold in the United States are standardized for content of the flavonoid silybin, a well-studied hepatoprotective agent. Silybin is believed to act primarily as a potent antioxidant and cellular protective agent. It has been shown to protect liver cells from a long list of negative effects resulting from iron, alcohol, carbon tetrachloride, radiation, acetaminophen, and ischemic injury.[40]

Silybin has been shown to be effective against a wide range of liver toxins. Most notably, it is known to be able to prevent liver destruction caused by poisoning from *Amanita phalloides* mushrooms (Fly Amanita, Death Cap). In a series of 41 mushroom poisonings treated within 48 hours with silymarin, there were no deaths.[41]

Silymarin has been well-evaluated in trials with alcoholic liver disease. At doses of 240 to 420mg per day, significant improvements in both histology (fibrosis) and serology (AST, ALT,

GGT, bilirubin, and alkaline phosphatase) are seen.[42–44] Silymarin also has demonstrated anti-inflammatory[45,46] and antifibrotic[47] effects in hepatic tissue.

For all of these reasons, researchers studying NASH have taken an interest in this herbal medicine. Currently, investigators at the Mayo Clinic Foundation are working on a phase II, open-label, pilot study of silymarin in patients with NASH. They will study 30 NASH patients taking doses of 600mg of silymarin standardized extract for two years. Until these results are available, it is not known if silymarin will prove effective for NASH as it has for other liver concerns.

## CONCLUSIONS

NAFLD is a common occurrence in patients presenting for WLS, which can prolong or complicate surgery. Modest preoperative weight reduction should be able to eliminate most concerns of liver size and retraction. Natural therapeutics may additionally benefit the health of patients by reducing associated risk factors, including inflammation, fibrosis, and hypertriglyceridemia. When looking at overall patient wellbeing, it may prove beneficial to selectively incorporate these therapies for use if indications are present.

## REFERENCES

1. Silverman JF, O'Brien KF, Long S, et al. Liver pathology in morbidly obese patients with and without diabetes. *Am J Gastroenterol* 1990;85:1349–55.
2. Spaulding L, Trainer T, Janiec D. Prevalence of nonalcoholic steatohepatitis in morbidly obese subjects undergoing gastric bypass. *Obes Surg* 2003;13(3):347–9.
3. Schwartz ML, Drew RL, Chazin-Caldie M. Laparoscopic Roux-en-Y gastric bypass: Preoperative determinants of prolonged operative times, conversion to open gastric bypasses, and postoperative complications. *Obes Surg* 2003;13:734–8.
4. Miller JC. Imaging and obese patients. *Radiol Rounds Mass General* 2005;3(7).
5. Dixon JB, Bhathal PS, O'Brien PE. Nonalcoholic fatty liver disease: predictors of nonalcoholic steatohepatitis and liver fibrosis in the severely obese. *Gastroenterology* 2001;121(1):91–100.
6. Scheen AJ, Luyckx FH. Obesity and liver disease. *Best Pract Res Clin Endocrinol Metab* 2002;16(4):703–16.
7. Blackburn GL, Mun EC. Effects of weight loss surgeries on liver disease. *Semin Liver Dis* 2004;24:371–9.
8. Tiikkainen M, Bergholm R, Vehkavaara S, et al. Effects of identical weight loss on body composition and features of insulin resistance in obese women with high and low liver fat content. *Diabetes* 2003;52:701–7.
9. Palmer M, Schaffner F. Effects of weight reduction on hepatic abnormalities in overweight patients. *Gastroenterology* 1990;99:1408–13.
10. Andersen T, Gluud C, Franzmann MB, Christoffersen P. Hepatic effects of dietary weight loss in morbidly obese subjects. *J Hepatol* 1991;12:224–9.
11. Marchesini G, Brizi M, Bianchi G, et al. Metformin in nonalcoholic steatohepatitis. *Lancet* 2001;358:893–4.
12. Neuschwander-Tetri BA, Brunt EM, Wehmeier KR, et al. Improved nonalcoholic steatohepatitis after 48 weeks of treatment with the PPAR-gamma ligand rosiglitazone. *Hepatology* 2003;38:1008–17.
13. Promrat K, Lutchman G, Uwaifo GI, et al. A pilot study of pioglitazone treatment for nonalcoholic steatohepatitis. *Hepatology* 2004;39:188–96.
14. Horlander J, Kwo P. Atorvastatin for the treatment of NASH. *Hepatology* 1997;26:544A.
15. Hatzitolios A, Savopoulos C, Lazaraki G, et al. Efficacy of omega-3 fatty acids, atorvastatin and orlistat in non-alcoholic fatty liver disease with dyslipidemia. *Indian J Gastroenterol* 2004;23(4):131–4.
16. Basaranoglu M, Acbay O, Sonsuz A. A controlled trial of gemfibrozil in the treatment of patients with nonalcoholic steatohepatitis. *J Hepatol* 1999;31:384.
17. Laurin J, Lindor KD, Crippin JS, et al. Ursodeoxycholic acid or clofibrate in the treatment of non-alcohol induced steatohepatitis:a pilot study. *Hepatology* 1996;23:1464–7.
18. Lindor KD, Kowdley KV, Heathcote EJ. Ursodeoxycholic acid for treatment of nonalcoholic steatohepatitis: Results of a randomized trial. *Hepatology* 2004;39(3):770–8.
19. Mehta K, Van Thiel DH, Shah N, Mobarhan S. Nonalcoholic fatty liver disease: Pathogenesis and the role of antioxidants. *Nutr Rev* 2002;60(9):289–93.
20. Vajro P, Mandato C, Franzese A, Ciccimarra E, Vitamin E treatment in pediatric obesity-related liver disease: A randomized study. *J Pediatr Gastroenterol Nutr* 2004;38(1):48–55.

21.     Hasegawa T, Yoneda M, Nakamura K, et al. Plasma transforming growth factor-b1 level and efficacy of --tocopherol in patients with non-alcoholic steatohepatitis: a pilot study. *Aliment Pharmacol Ther* 2001;15:1667–72.
22.     Harrison SA, Torgerson S, Hayashi P, et al. Vitamin E and vitamin C treatment improves fibrosis in patients with nonalcoholic steatohepatitis. *Am J Gastroenterol* 2003;98(11):2485–90.
23.     Adams LA, Angulo P. Vitamins E and C for the treatment of NASH: Duplication of results but lack of demonstration of efficacy. *Am J Gastroenterol* 2003;98(11):2348–50.
24.     Gulbahar O, Karasu Z, Ersoz G, et al. Treatment of nonalcoholic steatohepatitis with N-acetylcysteine. *Gastroenterology* 2000;118:A1444.
25.     Fulghesu AM, Ciampelli M, Muzj G, et al. N-acetyl-cysteine treatment improves insulin sensitivity in women with polycystic ovary syndrome. *Fertil Steril* 2002;77(6):1128–35.
26.     Threlkeld DS (ed). *Drug Facts and Comparisons.* St Louis, MO: Facts and Comparisons, 1997:1090–4.
27.     Saeian K, Curro K, Binion DG, et al. Plasma total homocysteine levels are higher in nonalcoholic steatohepatitis. *Hepatology* 1999;30:436A.
28.     Purohit V, Russo D. Role of S-adenosyl-L-methionine in the treatment of alcoholic liver disease: introduction and summary of the symposium. *Alcohol* 2002;27(3):151–4.
29.     Abdelmalek M, Angulo P, Jorgensen R, et al. Betaine, a promising new agent for patients with nonalcoholic steatohepatitis: results of a pilot study. *Am J Gastroenterol* 2001;96:2534–6.
30.     Arsenio L, Bodria P, Magnati G, et al. Effectiveness of long-term treatment with pantethine inpatients with dyslipidemia. *Clin Ther* 1986;8:537–45.
31.     Bertolini S, Donati C, Elicio N, et al. Lipoprotein changes induced by pantethine in hyperlipoproteinemic patients: Adults and children. *Int J Clin Pharmacol Ther Toxicol* 1986;24:630–7.
32.     Gaddi A, Descovich GC, Noseda G, et al. Controlled evaluation of pantethine, a natural hypolipidemic compound, in patients with different forms of hyperlipoproteinemia. *Atherosclerosis* 1984;50:73–83.
33.     Osono Y, Hirose N, Nakajima K, Hata Y. The effects of pantethine on fatty liver and fat distribution. *J Atheroscler Thromb* 2000;7:55–8.
34.     Covington MB. Omega-3 fatty acids. *Am Fam Physician* 2004;70(1):133–40.
35.     Kris-Etherton PM, Harris WS, Appel LJ. American Heart Association. Nutrition Committee. Fish consumption, fish oil, omega-3 fatty acids, and cardiovascular disease. *Circulation* 2002;106:2747–57.
36.     Griffen WO Jr., Bivins BA, Bell RM. The decline and fall of jejunoileal bypass. *Surg Gynecol Obstet* 1983;157:301–8.
37.     Freund HR. Abnormalities of liver function and hepatic damage associated with total pareteral nutrition. *Nutrition* 1991;7:1–5.
38.     Wigg AJ, Roberts-Thomson I, Dymock R, et al. The role of small intestinal bacterial overgrowth, intestinal permeability, endotoxaemia, and tumour necrosis factor-α in the pathogenesis of non-alcoholic steatohepatitis. *Gut* 2001;48:206–211.
39.     Luper S. A review of plants used in the treatment of liver disease: Part 1. *Altern Med Rev* 1998;3(6):410–21.
40.     Sabeel AI, Kurkus J, Lindholm T. Intensive hemodialysis and hemoperfusion treatment of Amanita mushroom poisoning. *Mycopathologia* 1995;131:107–14.
41.     Buzzelli G, Moscarella S, Giusti A, et al. A pilot study on the liver protective effect of silybin-phosphatidylcholine complex (1dB 1016) in chronic active hepatitis. *Int J Clin Pharmacol Ther Toxicol* 1993;31:456-60.
42.     Ferenci P, Dragosics B, Dittrich H, et al. Randomized controlled trial of silymarin treatment in patients with cirrhosis of the liver. *J Hepatol* 1989;9:105–13.
43.     Trinchet IC, Coste T, Levy VG. Treatment of alcoholic hepatitis with silymarin. A double-blind comparative study in 116 patients. *Gastroenterol Clin Biol* 1989;13:120-4
44.     Dehmlow C, Murawski N, de Groot H, et al.Scavenging of reactive oxygen species and inhibition of arachidonic acid metabolism by silibinin in human cells. *Life Sci* 1996;58:1591–600.
45.     Dehmlow C, Erhard J, de Groot H. Inhibition of Kupffer cell functions as an explanation for the hepatoprotective properties of silibinin. *Hepatology* 1996;23:749–54.
46.     Boigk G, Stroedter L, Herbst H. Silymarin collagen accumulation in early and advanced biliary fibrosis secondary to complete bile duct obliteration in rats. *Hepatology* 1997;26:643–9.

# PART 2:
# Postoperative Micronutrition

Currently, there is little agreement on exactly how to manage micronutrition in postoperative bariatric surgery patients. Perhaps the biggest question is: What constitutes adequate nutrition to prevent most cases of deficiency? As of the publication of this book, we do not have enough data on all nutrients for all procedures to accurately state what the ideal protocols should be. To the research-minded reader, reading this book should make it apparent that there is not only a need for more research on micronutrition in bariatrics, but also that weight loss surgery (WLS) offers a unique medical model for the advancement of overall knowledge of human nutrition.

Despite our current incomplete data, we can review the published literature to date, apply sound nutritional science, and make recommendations that are logical based on current understanding. If we can create a model for risk reduction, we can continue to improve and refine this model over time as our knowledge base grows.

The area of nutritional diagnosis will also be addressed for each nutrient. There are some nutrients for which medicine still does not agree on the best technique for identifying deficiencies; there is even some disagreement on normal ranges for some elements. I would remind clinicians that they are always working with real, live patients. It is important to look at the totality of what is presented. Patient-reported symptoms and signs found in physical exams may, in some instances, be the best confirmation of a problem. In the absence of hard laboratory data, the vast majority of essential nutrients are safe enough to use therapeutically in a clinical trial should other indications dictate

One area in which I receive many questions is the immediate postoperative days and weeks. Very few frank deficiencies are reported in this time, but some deficiencies, such as in thiamine or potassium, may develop acutely due to lack of intake or loss due to vomiting. One possible consideration in very early prevention would be to add an intravenous B-complex to the routine IVs being administered in the hospital. Intramuscular injection would also be an option. No protocols currently exist for this, and I am not personally aware of any bariatric programs engaged in this practice. It is, however, very safe. Premixes of vitamin complexes and trace elements are readily available for this purpose.

# CHAPTER 3

# Vitamin B1 (Thiamine)

Thiamine (also thiamin or vitamin B1) is part of the B complex vitamins. It was the very first compound identified as a vitamin, and thus retains its historical numerical place in the B vitamin family. Thiamine is found in a broad range of foods, from grains and nuts to pork and beans. It is thought to be easily absorbed by the body, except in special cases, such as surgical bypass of the upper small intestine and excess ingestion of ethanol. In the former case, some of the primary absorption sites for thiamine are missed, and in the latter ethanol actually blocks transport of thiamine from the gut into the body.

Dietary thiamine occurs in two forms: The free form that is found in plant products and the phosphorylated form found in animal products. Only free thiamine can be absorbed. When the phosphorylated form is ingested it can be acted upon by enzymes in the small intestine to free the thiamine from the phosphate group. Thiamine is primarily absorbed in the upper jejunum, with some uptake in the duodenum and ileum. Uptake occurs primarily via active absorption when intake is less than 5mg per day (the RDA is 1.5mg). At higher concentrations, passive diffusion increases as a percent of absorption. Thiamine is poorly stored in the body. Studies estimate that an adult will store approximately 30 milligrams of thiamine. Depletion can therefore occur rapidly if the supply is not continuously replenished.

Once absorbed into the body, thiamine is converted thiamin pyrophosphate (TPP), thiamin monophosphate (TMP), and thiamin triphosphate (TTP). This process is magnesium dependant, thus magnesium deficiency can contribute to the development of thiamine deficiency by reducing the amount of active thiamine available. The pyrophosphate (TPP) is considered to be the most important. TPP is a cofactor for several mitochondrial enzymes that contribute to the formation of acetyl-co A and succinyl-co A. Ultimately, this is a critical step in the production of energy from food. TPP also acts as a coenzyme to transketolase. Transketolase catalyzes the synthesis of the energy molecules ATP and GTP, the nucleic acids deoxyribonucleic acid (DNA) and ribonucleic acid (RNA), and other enzymes. TPP also appears to have a direct role in nerve conduction and muscle contraction, which would help to explain the potentially severe neurological symptoms that can occur in deficiency.

## DEFICIENCY

Thiamine has many important functions in the body but is especially critical for energy production and nerve transmission. For this reason Beriberi reflects problems related to high-energy need systems (the heart and brain) as well as nerve function. There are three classes of Beriberi: dry, wet, and cerebral (Wernicke-Korsakoff syndrome). Very mild deficiency presents with vague symptoms, such as fatigue, weakness, and difficulty concentrating. With dry Beriberi (which is most common), patients may complain of vomiting, loss of appetite, weakness, sleepiness, burning feet, calf and leg pain, abdominal pain, constipation, headache, and cramping. Peripheral polyneuropathy is also common, and this is one reason that a presumptive diagnosis of B12 deficiency should not be made in a gastric bypass patient in the absence of supportive lab data. The neuropathy of thiamine deficiency begins with fatigue and loss of sensation, pain, and "heaviness" in the legs. Then pretibial edema develops, along with glove-and-stocking paresthesias and difficulty with tasks such as climbing stairs and standing on one leg.[1] Burning pain, especially in the feet (although it can occur anywhere) is a hallmark symptom. If there is involvement of the brain (cerebral Beriberi), mental confusion can be a prominent symptom. While this can be severe enough to include symptoms of delusion, hallucination, or psychosis, more mild symptoms are confabulation, memory impairment, eye dysfunction such as double vision (due to optic neuropathy), inability to walk or stand, or waddling gait. Wet Beriberi presents with symptoms of congestive heart failure. This would not be expected in postoperative weight loss surgery patients as it most often results from excessive overeating of carbohydrates. To date, there are no published case reports of wet Beriberi after any form of WLS.

The true incidence of thiamine deficiency after weight loss surgery (WLS) is not known. Cases have been reported primarily with Roux-en-Y (RNY) procedures, but also with adjustable gastric banding (AGB) procedures and, in one instance, with an intragastric balloon (BIB) procedure. While the focus in published reports tends to be on Wernicke-Korsakoff syndrome, it is more likely that chronic deficiency, with much less dramatic symptoms, prevails.

Known risk factors for thiamine deficiency include poor intake, intestinal loss (primarily through vomiting), alcohol intake, eating disorders, and dialysis. The risk with WLS in most cases is tied to vomiting in the early weeks and months postoperatively. Additionally, decreased food intake, malabsorption, and adherence with nutrition recommendations all play a role.

The growing popularity of WLS has created a new axis for thiamine deficiency. While there are few reports in medical literature, thiamine has become a topic of increased interest and suspicion. In the case of WLS, especially gastric bypass, there may be more than one factor that plays into thiamine deficiency. The greatest risk appears to be in patients who develop vomiting or are unable to consume adequate amounts of food in the early weeks or months following surgery. This is compounded by a generally increased body demand for thiamine with any surgery, decreased food intake, and bypassing of key areas of vitamin uptake. Patients who undergo more rapid or greater-than-expected weight loss may also be at increased risk. There are also reports of chronic deficiency associated with alcohol intake, lack of supplementation, and onset of poor eating habits.[2] Subsequent development of anorexia or bulimia following WLS would be a significant risk for thiamine deficiency and has been reported in literature.[3]

| **NAMES FOR THIAMINE DEFICIENCY** |
|---|
| • **Beriberi**—The general name for thiamine deficiency. |
| • **Dry Beriberi**—Describes thiamine deficiency presenting with primary peripheral neuropathy. |
| • **Wet Beriberi**—Describes thiamine deficiency manifesting with primary cardiac symptoms and edema; may also have neuropathy. |
| • **Cerebral Beriberi**—Describes thiamine deficiency with primary central nervous symptom involvement (abnormal eye movement, gait disorder, apathy, confusion, profound memory changes). <br><br> -CNS impairment without amnesia is called Wernicke's encephalopathy <br> -CNS impairment with amnesia/ confabulation is called Wernicke-Korsakoff syndrome |
| • **Bariatric Beriberi**—Emerging term in bariatric medicine to describe patients with thiamine deficiency due to weight loss surgery. |

## LAB EVALUATION

Laboratory evaluation of thiamine status should be considered in patients with any suspect axis of deficiency (vomiting, anorexia, etc) or in those presenting with symptoms. It is

| CLINICAL DIAGNOSIS OF THIAMINE DEFICIENCY |
| --- |
| **Eyes**<br>• Reports of blurred vision or double vision<br>• Extraoccular palsy or paresis (Ophthalmoplegia)<br>• Weakness of cranial nerves III, IV, VI<br>• Nystagmus<br>• Optic neuropathy<br>• Retinal hemorrhages (rare) |
| **Ears**—Tinnitus |
| **Throat**<br>• Hoarseness, difficulty talking<br>• Difficulty swallowing<br>• Weakness of laryngeal nerve |
| **Face**<br>• Facial weakness<br>• Pallor |
| **Head**—Headache (especially in subclinical or chronic presentation) |
| **Mental status**<br>• Fatigue<br>• Poor concentration<br>• Memory loss or changes<br>• Retrograde amnesia<br>• Confabulation<br>• Depression<br>• Changes in concentration<br>• Apathy<br>• Dementia<br>• In advanced untreated disease, coma can occur |
| **Cardiovascular**<br>• Tachycardia<br>• Cardiomegaly<br>• ECG changes<br>    -prolonged QT<br>    -T-wave inversion<br>    -low voltage)<br>• Orthostatic hypotension<br>• Edema of the legs<br>• With advanced wet beriberi, congestive heart failure can occur |
| **Respiratory**—Shortness of breath (wet beriberi) |
| **Gastrointestinal**<br>• Nausea<br>• Vomiting<br>• Anorexia, loss of appetite<br>• Gas retention<br>• Severe constipation |
| **Genitourinary**<br>• Flaccid bladder<br>• Urinary retention |
| **Nerve**<br>• Burning feet<br>• Distal neuropathy that progresses proximally<br>• Numbness of toes<br>• Glove and stocking neuropathy<br>• Neuropathy characterized by pain, burning, heaviness<br>• Pre-tibial edema<br>• Clumsiness<br>• Diminished DTRs, especially patellar and Achilles<br>• Trophic changes (late disease)<br>• Difficulty standing from sit/squat<br>• Foot drop (late disease) |
| **Central**<br>• Waddling gait<br>• Cranial and vagal involvement (see symptom description in each system )<br>• Mental status changes<br>    -Cerebellar degeneration (late) with waddling gait, jerking of arms and legs, nystagmus |
| **Musculoskeletal**<br>• Leg weakness<br>• Hand weakness, loss of grip strength<br>• Weakness of dorsiflexion<br>• Cramping in calf muscles and feet<br>• Muscle atrophy (late disease) |

particularly important to evaluate thiamine deficiency in patients presenting with neuropathy and normal B12 status. Serum or whole blood thiamin will find moderate to severe deficiency, but is not appropriate to follow treatment as it responds too rapidly to supplementation and will correct before the deficiency itself is corrected. Erythrocyte or whole blood transketolase activity is the most accurate assessment of both deficiency and progress, but may be hard to obtain through some labs. Urinary excretion appears to be relatively accurate. Pyruvate levels below 1mg/dL are also considered to be reliable.[3] One may also want to check TSH (to rule out hyperthyroidism as a cause of thiamine deficiency), serum folate (low folate is an indirect cause of thiamine deficiency), and liver enzymes (to rule out occult alcohol abuse).

Other diagnosis for thiamine deficiency may include nerve conduction studies (NCS) and electromyography (EMG), which are primarily of use in evaluating the severity of a neuropathy. NCS typically reveal decreases in both sensory nerve action potentials and compound muscle action potentials. Conduction velocity of both motor and sensory nerves may be slowed and distal latency somewhat prolonged. EMG may reveal signs of peripheral demyelination and denervation, especially in the lower extremity.

## TREATMENT

Treatment of thiamine deficiency should be implemented rapidly with a confirmed diagnosis. Given the safe, non-toxic nature of thiamine, it is also reasonable to begin therapy in presumed cases without a confirmed diagnosis. In fact, improvement with therapy may be the most rapid

indication of a deficiency
as thiamine mononitrate
can be initiated with 50
When emesis subsides,
moved to a 50 to 100m
fully resolve. If neurop
resolution is typically
thiamine therapy to t
thiamine does not cc
critical because absc
acid. Additionally, a
to its active form; t
on Magnesium).

As discussed in
preoperatively. Ba
deficiency could
little to no nutrit
patients are disc
care be aware c

## INTERACTIONS

Aside from these food interactions, there ar
Loop diuretics, such as furosemide (Lasix®)
phenytoin (Dilantin®) appear to disrupt th
the chemotherapeutic agent, 5-Flurouc
thiamine status, although the implica
mentioned in the section on treatn
B12, folate, and magnesium.

## CONCLUSIONS

Thiamine is a critica
acute symptoms in c
can be vague and r
question that ha
status should
evidence to
between
those
clini

## PREVENTION AND MAINTE...

Beyond resolution of deficiency, the exact amount of thiamine
status after WLS is not known. In the absence of vomiting, anorexia, eating disor
alcoholism, it would be reasonable to assume that the Daily Value (DV) of 1.5mg should be
adequate for most. However, because the primary absorptive sites are bypassed with some
bariatric procedures, and dietary sources may be diminished, more could be necessary. Again,
thiamine is very safe, so higher levels should not be harmful. Most multivitamin formulations
provide at least the DV of thiamine. The Food and Nutrition Board of the Institute of
Medicine has not set a tolerable upper level (UL) because no evidence of oral toxicity has
been seen even with doses as high as 200mg taken for long periods of time. Intravenous
thiamine has been known to produce rare anaphylactic reactions.

Thiamine is widespread in foods; however, fortified grains are the richest and most
common source in most diets. Legumes, nuts, and pork are also good sources. Some foods
also contain anti-thiamine factors (ATFs). ATFs act to oxidize dietary thiamine in the
digestive system and render it inactive. They are commonly found in coffee (including
decaffeinated) and black tea. Some polyphenols, such as those in blueberries and the cabbage
family, may also act as ATFs. Raw or fermented fish contains the enzyme thiaminase, which
destroys thiamine. This is not a concern in cooked fish, since heat inactivates this enzyme.
Additionally, chlorine compounds that may be found in drinking water can destroy thiamine
with prolonged contact. For example, rice cooked in chlorinated water may have one-third
less thiamine than rice cooked in filtered or distilled water.[4] Due to these unique interactions
of thiamine and foods, it may be wise to counsel thiamine deficient patients or at-risk patients
about these substances.

e some known drug interactions with thiamine.
, increase urinary excretion of thiamine, and
iamine metabolism, resulting in low levels, as does
l. Oral contraceptives and antacids may also alter
ions with these drugs are not well understood. As
ent, thiamine interacts with other nutrients, including B6,

nutrient that can clearly be a deficiency risk in WLS patients. While
ses of rapid onset may be easily identified, chronic or subacute deficiency
ay not be obvious from physical signs and reported symptoms alone. One
recently arisen in the bariatric community is whether testing for thiamine
be part of routine labs. At this writing, there does not appear to be sufficient
support this, although some programs are requiring a screening test at some point
and 6 months postoperative. Preoperative screening may be advisable to identify
atients who might be at the greatest risk of early-onset deficiency. It is advisable for
cians following the care of WLS patients to be aware of the signs and symptoms that would
rt them to testing and intervention.

## REFERENCES

1. Sewell AR, Recht, LD. *Nutritional Neuropathy* http://www.emedicine.com/med/topic221.htm, Access date: 25 May 2005.
2. Grace DM, Alfieri MA, Leung FY. Alcohol and poor compliance as factors in Wernicke's encephalopathy diagnosed 13 years after gastric bypass. *Can J Surg* 1998;41(5):389–92.
3. Bonne OB, Bashi R, Berry EM. Anorexia nervosa following gastroplasty in the male: Two cases. *Int J Eat Disord* 1996;19(1):105–8.
4. Yagi N, Itokawa Y. Cleavage of thiamine by chlorine in tap water. *J Nutr Sci Vitaminol* (Tokyo) 1979;25(4):281–7.

# CHAPTER 4

# Folate (Folic Acid, Pteroylglutamic Acid)

Folate is a B vitamin that has several coenzyme functions in the human body. The two primary reactions for which folate is critical are the synthesis of nucleic acids and the synthesis of methionine from homocysteine. The latter reaction also requires B12 (see Chapter 5). A shortage of either nutrient may result in elevated homocysteine levels, which is discussed later. Folate is also used in histidine metabolism (specifically in the generation of glutamate from formiminoglutamic acid [FIGLU]). Finally, the synthesis of purines and pyrimidines require folate derivatives. Because these substances are important to cell division, folate shortages can affect new cell growth. The fact that folate plays a critical role in nucleic acid synthesis as well as in cell division explains why some problems occur when folate status is not optimal. Birth defects, especially neural tube defects, are highly correlated to folate deficiency. Low folate may also contribute to heart and limb malformations. Some cancers, especially colon and breast, are associated with folate deficiency, perhaps because of flawed deoxyribonucleic acid (DNA) repair. In the case of colon cancer, the role of folate in rapid cell division may also come into play, as enterocytes are short-lived and known to be sensitive to folate status.

Folate is primarily absorbed in the jejunum (more proximal than distal) and is somewhat absorbed in the duodenum. Absorption in the ileum is insignificant.[1] Research indicates that there are both passive and active absorption systems. It appears that passive diffusion only occurs after the transport protein involved in active transport is saturated.[2] Folates in foods and folic acid in dietary supplements are chemically different from each other in ways that influence absorption. This is because folate in food must be hydrolyzed by brush border enzymes before being absorbed from the gut. The hydrolysis process is zinc dependent; thus, zinc deficiency can contribute to folate deficiency. Folic acid in fortified foods and dietary supplements actually have much greater bioavailability for this reason. Furthermore, folic acid taken on an empty stomach is significantly better absorbed than that taken with food (or fortified into food). Because these differences are significant and can be calculated, the Institute of Medicine has introduced the Dietary Folate Equivalent (DFE) as a new unit of measurement for folates. These units are calculated as follows:

- 1mcg of folate in food provides 1mcg of DFE.
- 1mcg of folic acid taken in a fortified food or taken with a meal provides 1.7mcg of DFE.
- 1mcg of folic acid as a supplement taken on an empty stomach provides 2mcg of DFE.

This essentially means that 400mcg of folate from a dietary supplement taken on an empty stomach is equal to 800mcg of folate naturally occurring in a food. Because the recommended daily allowance (RDA) is now based on DFE, calculating the daily folate intake of patients who have undergone weight loss surgery (WLS) is important. Based on the DFE, patients with folate deficiency have the best opportunity for absorption when taking folate alone on an empty stomach.

Once absorbed, most folate is transported to the liver and approximately half remains there in storage. In the liver, folates can be converted to polyglutamate derivatives for transport throughout the body. The primary circulating form is 5-methyltetrahydrofolate. In individuals taking folic acid, this form is also found in circulation. Circulating folate is about two-thirds bound and one-third unbound.

## DEFICIENCY

Folate deficiency is associated with neural tube defects, cardiovascular disease, and some cancers. These conditions are not necessarily useful clinical indications, but they underscore the serious nature of deficiency and the impact on long-term health. Since 1998, the US has had the folic acid fortification program. This was put into place because the 1994 National Health and Nutrition Examination Survey (NHANES III) showed that most female Americans did not consume adequate folic acid to protect themselves in their

## WHEN FOLATE IS TOO HIGH

In general, elevated folate is probably a sign that a patient has recently taken a dietary supplement containing folic acid. However, there are other interesting causes. Some of these include false elevation from sample hemolysis, pernicious anemia, rare false elevation with iron deficiency, small intestinal bacterial overgrowth (SIBO) and blind loop syndrome.

Blind loop syndrome can cause bacterial overgrowth in the small intestine and is known to occur with procedures like Roux-en-y (RNY) or Billroth II surgery for stomach ulcers. SIBO is also known to occur in the short bowel from all causes. In some individuals, bacteria or abnormal flora may begin to overgrow in the bypassed portion of the intestine, causing weight loss, nausea, fatty/frothy stools, bloating, abdominal pain, loss of appetite, and alterations of nutrient absorption. SIBO is also a cause of lactose intolerance. Symptoms may be intermittent and overlap with common symptoms produced by surgery, which may make them hard to identify. As discussed earlier in this book, significant overgrowth of bacteria in the obsolete JIB procedure was known to be responsible for complications, including inflammatory arthritis, dermatitis, malaise, and serious liver pathology (including liver failure).[1]

The most common bacteria that overgrow in these syndromes are streptococci, bacteroides, *E. coli*, and lactobacilli.[2] While some of these normally occur, in SIBO or blind loop syndrome, they may be present at many hundreds to thousands of times above normal levels. Additionally, overgrowth of abnormal flora or bacteria can create problems of toxicity, directly damaging the intestinal lining or, if absorbed, the liver.

Blind loop syndrome is thought to contribute to deficiency of vitamin D, iron, and B12. Since these deficiencies are common in WLS, they are not distinct. However, it has been noted that the combined finding of elevated serum folate and low serum B12 is indicative of SIBO with or without blind loop syndrome. This is because the abnormal bacteria can synthesize folate, and when they make enough, it will be absorbed into systemic circulation. It is usually more common to see both nutrients at normal or low levels in WLS patients. Therefore, this finding may indicate the need for further screening to rule out this complication.

Tests to confirm diagnosis include barium x-ray, hydrogen, or D-xylose breath testing. Endoscopy with aspiration is a very accurate diagnostic tool, but may not be possible after WLS. Antibiotics are a common treatment, as is nutritional support (which most patients already undergo). Additionally, it may be wise to consider reinoculation of the gastrointestinal tract with healthy flora following antibiotic therapy. This could include yogurt with live cultures or a probiotic supplement, such as *Lactobacillus casei*, *Lactobacillus reuterii*, or *Lactobacillus GG*.

### REFERENCES

1. Griffen Jr, WO, Bivins BA, Bell RM. The decline and fall of jejunoileal bypass. *Surg Gynecol Obstet* 1983;157:301–8.
2. Bouhnik Y, Alain S, Attar A, et al. Bacterial populations contaminating the upper gut in patients with small intestinal bacterial overgrowth syndrome. *Am J Gastroenterol* 1999;94:1327–31.

childbearing years. However, the products that are enriched under this program (cereal, enriched pasta, bread, waffles) are largely foods that many WLS patients are instructed to avoid after surgery.

Folic acid deficiency does not have any remarkable clinical features of its own. Most of the symptoms are those that overlap with B12 deficiency, with gastrointestinal disorders

| CLINICAL DIAGNOSIS OF FOLATE DEFICIENCY |
| --- |
| **Eyes** <br>• Congenital eye defects <br>• Optic neuropathy |
| **Throat** <br>• Gingivitis <br>• Canker sores <br>• Glossitis (swollen tongue) |
| **Face** <br>• Pallor <br>• Possible hyperpigmentation or blotchy pigment in dark-skinned individuals |
| **Head** <br>• Lightheadedness <br>• Faintness |
| **Mental status** <br>• Fatigue <br>• Poor concentration <br>• Memory loss or changes <br>• Retrograde amnesia <br>• Confabulation <br>• Depression <br>• Changes in concentration <br>• Apathy <br>• Dementia <br>• Coma (can occur in advanced untreated disease) |
| **Cardiovascular** <br>• Palpitations <br>• Angina <br>• With high homocysteine – increased risk for stroke and MI |
| **Gastrointestinal** <br>• Anorexia, loss of appetite <br>• Hepatomegaly <br>• Splenomegaly (if anemia is present) <br>• Diarrhea |
| **Nervous System – symptoms are identical to B12 deficiency** <br>• Central and Peripheral Neuropathy <br>• Isolated neuropathy – 25% <br>• Neuropathy + Myelopathy – 40% <br>• Neurological exam may be normal in some patients <br>• Glove and stocking neuropathy – legs affected before arms – rarely all limbs <br>• Pins and needles, coldness, numbness, constricted or swollen feelings are often noted <br>• Sharp, lancing pains <br>• Loss of Achilles reflex – 50% <br>• Patellar reflex may be hyper at first then lost <br>• Positive Babinski sign <br>• Positive Romberg (relatively common) <br>• Positive Hoffman's sign (late) <br>• Decreased vibratory sense <br>• Decreased pinprick, light touch, and temperature sensation (ascends in pattern of neuropathy) <br>• Wide gait <br>• Restless leg syndrome |
| **Musculoskeletal** <br>• Distal muscular atrophy <br>• Sensation of tightness in fingers and toes <br>• Limb weakness |
| **Hematologic** <br>• MCV >100 <br>• Macro-ovalocytosis <br>• Anisocytosis <br>• Poikilocytosis <br>• Irregular platelets <br>• Polynuclear lymphocytes |
| **Legs** <br>• Ankle edema <br>• See Musculoskeletal and Nervous System Symptoms |
| **Other** <br>• In women, repeat spontaneous abortion <br>• Cancer of the colon <br>• Breast and cervical cancer |

(such as Celiac disease) that have a high prevalence of folate deficiency, and with anemia.

Folate deficiency can present as fatigue, weakness, faintness, irritability, depression, loss of appetite, diarrhea (which may also be the cause), forgetfulness, canker sores, sore swollen tongue (glossitis), palpitations, and angina. Physical examination may show ankle edema, hepatomegaly, splenomegaly, and areas of skin hyperpigmentation.

Older texts may claim that folate deficiency does not cause neuropathy; however, although neuropathy is more common in combined deficiency states, isolated cases have been reported.[3] Neuropathy is also associated with drug-induced folate deficiency.[4] The neurological symptoms of folate deficiency can be identical to B12 deficiency with dementia and sensorimotor polyneuropathy. Restless leg syndrome has also been reported.

Prevalence of folate deficiency after WLS is documented to some degree with all procedures. Reported levels of deficiency range from close to 40 percent[5] to as low as one percent.[6] Elevated homocysteine levels are also reported after all types of procedures.[7-10] Mallory and MacGregor suggested that the large discrepancies were a measure of adherence with a multivitamin, which appears to be a reasonable assumption based on later data.[11]

## LAB EVALUATION

Several methods exist for the evaluation of folate status. Megaloblastic anemia of folate deficiency is identical to that of B12 deficiency and cannot be used for definitive diagnosis. Likewise, while hypersegmentation of neutrophils is the earliest hematologic change found with folate deficiency, B12 deficiency can also create this finding. Serum folate levels are commonly used, but are mostly reflective of very recent dietary intake and not of tissue levels. In fact, one can see megaloblastic anemia of folate deficiency with normal serum folate.[12] Red blood cell/erythrocyte folate levels have become a much more stable marker of true folate status. However, if anemia is present, low red blood cells (RBC) folate will still not rule out the presence of B12 deficiency. In B12 deficiency, one can find low RBC folate, and normal or even elevated RBC folate. Moreover, if one doses folate at high enough levels in a patient with B12 deficiency, the anemia can be corrected while the B12 deficiency remains. For these reasons, is it important to check B12 status together with folate status.

A variety of other markers are sometimes evaluated with folate deficiency. As with B12 deficiency, homocysteine levels will rise. FIGLU excretion, deoxyuridine suppression (dUST), and folate excretion are all available, but are mostly experimental and their true utility in clinical nutrition is not yet apparent. For now, the combination of RBC folate together with serum B12 offers the most useful assessment. Homocysteine is also a great functional marker to follow in recovery. A normal methylmalonic acid level with an elevated homocysteine level also confirms the diagnosis of folate deficiency and rules out B12 deficiency.

## TREATMENT

With frank symptomatic folate deficiency, a dose of 3 to 5mg of folic acid can be given between meals until RBC levels and homocysteine levels return to normal range and anemia is corrected. With mild deficiency, consider a lower level of 1mg (1000mcg). Continuing supplementation of B12 during this time is a good idea, even if deficiency has been ruled out, since these nutrients are so important to each other. If the patient has difficulty eating or experiences ongoing diarrhea, folic acid can be given as an intramuscular injection. The typical dose is 1cc (providing 1000mcg), until the deficiency reverses or the patient can tolerate oral dosing. In particularly difficult cases of hyperhomocysteinemia that do not reverse with normal folate, B12, and possibly B6 supplementation, folinic acid can be given. Folinic acid, also known as 5-formyl tetrahydrofolate (leukovorin), is an activated form of folate that is more "potent" and more bioavailable than folic acid (it is also much more expensive). This form is often used to rescue bone marrow in patients taking methotrexate. While very high doses (25–125mg) are sometimes used in chemotherapy patients, a dose for difficult homocysteine would be more in the range of 1mg to 5mg.

Folic acid deficiency usually corrects in 2 to 3 months from the time therapy is initiated. Female patients should guard against pregnancy during folate deficiency.

## PREVENTION AND MAINTENANCE

There is reasonable evidence that multivitamins containing 400 to 800mcg of folate are protective for most WLS patients. Mallory and MacGregor found that absence of folate deficiency was highly correlated with multivitamin adherence.[6] This is good to know not only because it gives clinicians a way to check for suspected nonadherence, but it may serve to help motivate patients to continue with multivitamin supplementation long-term.

Because many WLS patients avoid the foods that are fortified under the Folic Acid Food

Fortification Program of 1998, they should be advised of other food sources of folate. Good sources include oranges and orange juice, green vegetables, peanuts, peas, legumes, sprouts, liver, and soybeans.

## EXCESS AND TOXICITY

The Institute of Medicine lists 1000mcg as the tolerable upper limit (UL) for folic acid, and limits over-the-counter (OTC) supplements to 800mcg. This is not because of toxicity, but rather because high-dose folate can mask B12 deficiency. In the absence of B12 deficiency, folate is safe at almost unlimited doses.

## INTERACTIONS

Most of the interactions with medications for folate are called "beneficial interactions"— meaning that the combined effect is better than the drug alone. This is true with some antidepressants (SSRIs), diuretics, and birth control. Anticonvulsants should not be taken together with folic acid unless under physician supervision. At levels of 800mcg and above, folate may lower seizure threshold.[13] Folic acid should also be avoided with methotrexate unless advised by a physician.

As mentioned earlier, zinc deficiency can impair folate absorption from food by decreasing the activity of brush-border enzymes. These specific enzymes are also inhibited by some foods, including oranges, cabbage, cruciferous vegetables, and many legumes. This does not apply to folate in dietary supplements, which does not have to undergo hydrolysis to be absorbed. Some animal studies have shown that folate may also somewhat impair zinc absorption when taken together, but studies in humans have not confirmed any impact.

Finally, B12 and folate have a very close, synergistic relationship. The enzyme methionine synthase requires both B12 and folate. In the absence of adequate B12, N5-methyl THF (which is required for producing methionine from homocysteine) cannot be recycled back to THF. Thus the overall folate pool is reduced and methylation reactions are impaired. This is called the "folate trap."

## CONCLUSION

Folic acid deficiency should be rare in WLS patients who adhere with multivitamin therapy. Knowing this, clinicians can utilize measurements of folate to help assess adherence. For this reason, including RBC folate as part of the annual lab work is a good idea. It is also important to assess folate in women who are or desire to become pregnant.

## REFERENCES

1.    Hepner GW, Booth CC, Cowan J, et al. Absorption of crystalline folic acid in man. *Lancet* 1968;2:302–6.
2.    Halstead CH. Intestinal absorption and malabsorption of folates. *Ann Rev Med* 1980;31:79–87.
3.    Lossos A, Argov Z, Ackerman Z, Abramsky O. Peripheral neuropathy and folate deficiency as the first sign of Crohn's disease. *J Clin Gastroenterol* 1991;13(4):442–4.
4.    Perry TE. Folate responsive neuropathy. *Presse Med* 1994;23(3):131–7.
5.    Halverson JD. Micronutrient deficiencies after gastric bypass for morbid obesity. *Am Surg* 1986;52(11):594–8.

6.  Mallory GN, Macgregor AM. Folate status following gastric bypass surgery (the great folate mystery). *Obes Surg* 1991;1(1):69–72.

7.  Sheu WH, Wu HS, Wang CW, et al. Elevated plasma homocysteine concentrations six months after gastroplasty in morbidly obese subjects. *Intern Med* 2001;40(7):584–8.

8.  Brolin RE, Leung M. Survey of vitamin and mineral supplementation after gastric bypass and biliopancreatic diversion for morbid obesity. *Obes Surg* 1999;9(2):150–4.

9.  Hocking MP, Davis GL, Franzini DA, Woodward ER. Long-term consequences after jejunoileal bypass for morbid obesity. *Dig Dis Sci* 1998;43(11):2493–9.

10. Dixon JB, Dixon ME, O'Brien PE. Elevated homocysteine levels with weight loss after Lap-Band surgery: Higher folate and vitamin B12 levels required to maintain homocysteine level. *Int J Obes Relat Metab Disord* 2001;25(2):219–27.

11. Brolin RE, Gorman JH, Gorman RC, et al. Are vitamin B12 and folate deficiency clinically important after Roux-en-Y gastric bypass? *J Gastrointest Surg* 1998;2(5):436–42.

12. Hoffbrand AV, Newcombe BF, Molin DL. Method of assay of red cell folate activity and the value of the assay as a test for folate deficiency. *J Clin Pathol* 1966;19(1):17–28.

13. Guidolin L, Vignoli A, Canger R. Worsening in seizure frequency and severity in relation to folic acid administration. *Eur J Neurol* 1998;5:301.

# CHAPTER 5

# Vitamin B12 (Cobalamin)

Vitamin B12 was first discovered in the late 1940s as a treatment for pernicious anemia. It is unique among the B-complex vitamins in that it contains a metal ion, cobalt. The alternate name for this vitamin, cobalamin, reflects this unique feature.

B12 has several critical roles in human nutrition. On its own, B12 is required for the creation of cellular energy from dietary fats and proteins. It is a cofactor in the creation of the Krebs cycle intermediate succinyl-CoA, which is required for the production of hemoglobin. For this reason, deficiency of B12 can lead to hemoglobin-deficient anemia. B12's other functions are mostly performed in conjunction with folic acid. Together, these nutrients are used in the synthesis of methionine and S-adenosylmethionine (SAMe). SAMe donates methyl groups for the synthesis of deoxyribonucleic acid (DNA) and ribonucleic acid (RNA). It also donates a methyl group for the recycling of homocysteine back to methionine.[1] Thus, a shortage of B12, leading to a shortage of SAMe, can result in a toxic build-up of homocysteine.

Less well understood is the role of B12 in the health of myelin and the nervous system. While we know that deficiency will result in myelin degradation and a well-recognized neuropathy, the mechanism behind this has not been fully elucidated. One possible etiology is based on deficiency of SAMe. SAMe is important for the production and maintenance of myelin, especially for the creation of structural phospholipids. SAMe is also used in the production of the neurotransmitters dopamine, norepinephrine, and serotonin, which may help explain why symptoms of depression and cognitive impairment are sometimes reported with low B12.

## ABSORPTION

Absorption of B12 from normal dietary sources is an intricate process that is the most complex of the recognized essential nutrients. B12 from food is separated from protein by the action of both hydrochloric acid and pepsin. It then binds to a protein from saliva called protein R. This complex leaves the stomach where it is digested by pancreatic enzymes. B12 then binds to intrinsic factor (IF) in the upper small intestine. IF is a glycoprotein excreted by parietal cells in the stomach. Finally, the IF-bound B12 is absorbed at special receptor sites in the ileum. This process accounts for 99 percent of B12 absorption. Approximately one percent of B12 can be absorbed by passive diffusion if no IF is present.[2] In addition, B12 can be reabsorbed in the gut after being excreted in bile. This process is called enterohepatic recirculation. B12 excreted through bile must also bind to IF to be absorbed.

## STORAGE

Unlike most water-soluble vitamins, the body stores a significant amount of vitamin B12. Most storage is in the liver, but the heart, spleen, kidneys, and brain also store vitamin B12. Since the total average body storage is 2 to 10mg, and the daily usage is about 2.5mcg, it can take a long time for B12 deficiency to present even in a complete absence of intake. This is important to keep in mind when evaluating WLS patients, and in enforcing the need for long-term nutritional follow-up.

## RISK FOR DEFICIENCY WITH WLS

In the general population, B12 deficiency is estimated to occur in 3 to 30 percent of adults. The incidence of deficiency increases markedly with age, and studies suggest that at age 65, 15 percent of the population is deficient. Outside of intestinal surgery, which we will address specifically here, other causes of deficiency include pernicious anemia (which affects up to 2% of adults and accounts for greater than 70% of reported deficiencies), atrophic gastritis, infection with *Helicobacter pylori*, veganism, alcoholism, fad dieting, poor nutrient intake (especially in the elderly), diseases of the terminal ileum, HIV infection, multiple sclerosis, and the use of some prescription medications like proton pump inhibitors. There are likely multiple

| SERUM B12 SCREENING TEST | |
|---|---|
| **B12 Level** | **Action** |
| • Below 100 | • Treat for B12 deficiency |
| • Between 100 and 400 | • Test homocysteine and MMA<br>– If both are high, treat for B12 deficiency and give folate<br>– If homocysteine WNL, MMA are high, treat for B12 deficiency<br>– If MMA WNL, homocysteine are high, test for folate deficiency |
| • Above 400 | • Re-test in 1 year or if symptoms occur |

reasons for B12 deficiency following WLS. General risk factors, as stated previously, may be predisposing issues. One study in Roux-en-y (RNY) surgery patients found a 25-percent incidence of active *Helicobacter pylori* infection, and an 82-percent incidence of gastritis.[3] Maldigestion due to loss of stomach functions and malabsorption due to loss of IF are clear problems. Finally, increased physiologic demand during rapid weight loss may be a factor, especially in restrictive procedures.

Because of the multiple roles of the stomach in B12 digestion and absorption, gastrointestinal surgery is a significant risk for deficiency. Loss of hydrochloric acid, gastric churning, pepsin, and IF are all causes of B12 malnutrition. Both partial and total gastrectomy are considered to be serious risks for B12 deficiency—this includes gastric bypass, duodenal switch (DS), and gastric sleeves. However, gastric banding has also been shown to produce a conditional increase in B12 requirements.

## MALABSORPTIVE AND COMBINED PROCEDURES

The greatest risk for B12 deficiency in WLS is with malabsorptive or combined procedures. B12 deficiency is reported to occur in one-third of postoperative patients after one year and may increase thereafter depending on nutritional adherence. Some studies have shown incidence as high as 70 percent.[4] Published data estimates a 37-percent B12 deficiency rate after RNY and an 11-percent rate after DS. Risk with gastric sleeve has never been studied. Nonetheless, partial gastrectomy itself is a known risk factor for B12 malnutrition, having been demonstrated in procedures for ulcer and gastric cancer.

## RESTRICTIVE PROCEDURES

Much less is known about B12 status following restrictive procedures. One small study evaluated levels of B12, folate, and iron after vertical banded gastroplasty (VBG) and found a 10 percent deficiency level after one year.[5] Adjustable gastric banding (AGB) has been shown to produce conditionally increased needs for vitamin B12. A control-matched study of nearly

| CLINICAL DIAGNOSIS OF B12 DEFICIENCY |
| --- |
| **Eyes** <br> • Decreased visual acuity <br> • Field defects <br> • Optic atrophy—wasting of or pallid optic disc may be visualized in late disease <br> • Nystagmus <br> • Small pupils |
| **Ears** <br> • Sensorineural deafness (rare) |
| **Throat/Mouth** <br> • Glossitis <br> • Burning of lips and mouth <br> • Patchy erythema in the mouth |
| **Face** <br> • Pallor <br> • Possible hyperpigmentation—or blotchy pigment in dark-skinned individuals |
| **Head** <br> • Lightheadedness <br> • Vertigo <br> • Premature graying of hair |
| **Mental status** <br> • Fatigue <br> • Depression <br> • Mild dementia <br> • General cognitive decline <br> • Blunted affect <br> • Emotional lability <br> • Disorientation <br> • Psychosis <br> • Delusions |
| **Cardiovascular** <br> • Tachycardia <br> • Palpitations <br> • Angina <br> • Cardiomegaly <br> • With high homocysteine—increased risk for stroke and MI |
| **Gastrointestinal** <br> • Anorexia, loss of appetite <br> • Glossitis <br> • Hepatosplenomegaly (if anemia is present) <br> • Sensation of constriction in the abdomen <br> • Mild jaundice is possible |
| **Nervous System** <br> • Central and peripheral neuropathy <br> • Isolated neuropathy, 25% <br> • Neuropathy + myelopathy, 40% <br> • Neurological exam may be normal in some patients <br> • Glove and stocking neuropathy—legs affected before arms, rarely all limbs; Pins and needles, coldness, numbness, constricted or swollen feelings are often noted; Sharp, lancing pains <br> • Loss of Achilles reflex, 50% <br> • Patellar reflex may be hyper at first then lost <br> • Positive Babinski sign <br> • Positive Romberg (relatively common) <br> • Positive Hoffman's sign (late) <br> • Decreased vibratory sense <br> • Decreased pinprick, light touch and temperature sensation (ascends in pattern of neuropathy) <br> • Wide gait |
| **Musculoskeletal** <br> • Distal muscular atrophy <br> • Sensation of tightness in fingers and toes <br> • Limb weakness |
| **Hematologic** <br> • MCV >100 <br> • Macro-ovalocytosis <br> • Anisocytosis <br> • Poikilocytosis <br> • Irregular platelets <br> • Polynuclear lymphocytes |

300 patients examined serum B12, folate, and homocysteine levels over a two-year period following AGB placement.[6] Those undergoing weight loss had significant elevations of total homocysteine levels compared to controls. While low levels of serum B12 or folate explained 35 percent of the elevations, researchers found that in the remainder of cases, higher baseline levels of these nutrients were required to maintain normal homocysteine levels. The study concluded that "there is an altered dose-response relationship with higher serum B(12) and folate levels required to maintain recommended [homocysteine] levels. Patients losing weight have significant health benefits; however, they may be at greater risk of vascular events or fetal abnormality in association with raised [homocysteine] levels.[6]"

# EVALUATION OF B12 NUTRITION

**Signs and symptoms of deficiency.** Patients may or may not report symptoms of vitamin B12 deficiency. Early signs of nervous system involvement may be vague or transient and may go unnoticed by patients for an extended period of time. Other early signs, such as fatigue, weakness, shortness of breath, and loss of appetite, are generally quite common in WLS patients and, unless they are profound, are not specific enough to clearly indicate a problem with B12 nutrition.

As deficiency progresses, symptoms indicative of peripheral nervous system or spinal cord involvement are most often those reported in a clinical visit. On average, three quarters of B12-deficient patients will present with neurologic manifestations. The classic triad of symptoms is the combined presentation of weakness, paresthesia, and sore tongue. Paresthesia is usually the

## COMPARING THIAMINE DEFICIENCY TO B12 DEFICIENCY

| Sign/Symptom | Thiamine | B12 |
|---|---|---|
| Onset | Usually in first 6 months, but can be any time | Usually after 6 months, but can be any time |
| Reported incidence | Unknown, but reported with all procedures | Approximately 37% after RNY, 11% after DS, also reported after AGB |
| Vomiting | Common | Not a symptom |
| Loss of appetite | Yes | Yes |
| Calf/leg/foot pain | Yes | Numbness and paresthesias is more common |
| Paresthesias | Yes, often with pain, burning, and heaviness. Usually starts in lower extremity. Glove and stocking distribution is common. Burning feet is common. | Yes, glove and stocking, starts most often in lower extremity, pins and needles, coldness, numbness, constricted or swollen feelings are often noted. |
| Atrophy | Yes—dorsum of feet (late sign) | Muscle wasting can occur |
| Weakness | Yes | Most common if anemia develops |
| Sore tongue | No | Yes |
| Pre-tibial edema | Yes | No |
| Loss of balance | Yes | Yes |
| Dementia | Yes, with Korsakoff's syndrome | Often first symptom, clinically identical to other dementias |
| Depression | No | Yes |
| Clumsiness | Yes | Yes, mostly in hands |
| Gait abnormality | Yes, waddling gait | Yes, wide/slow gait; a "slapping" gait |
| Cramping | Common in feet, calves | Not described |
| Eye dysfunction | Yes—blurred/double vision, optic neuropathy | Decreased visual acuity and field defects |
| Ear/hearing | Tinnitus may occur | Sensorineural deafness may occur, but rare |
| Autonomic | Yes—bladder, bowel, hypotension | N/A |
| Psychosis | Yes – can be early sign | Yes—but late sign |
| Memory impairment | Yes—can be acute and profound or chronic (see dementia); anterograde | General cognitive decline may be seen. |
| Reflexes | Patellar and Achilles reflexes are decreased | Patellar may be absent, 50% have loss of Achilles reflex, hyper-reflexia is rare, Babinski may be positive |
| Vibration | N/A | Decreased |
| Anemia | Only described in genetic deficiency | Yes, megaloblastic with decreased hematocrit and increased MCV |
| Heart | CHF with wet beriberi. May see tachycardia if vagus nerve is involved. | Cardiomegaly can be a late sign that can occur with anemia. May also see palpitations, angina, tachycardia. |
| Other | Vagus nerve involvement with tachycardia, hoarseness, dysphagia, difficulty talking, trophic changes (shiny skin, hair loss in dermatomes) | Glossitis; occasional hyperpigmentation of skin; decreased temperature sensation |

symptom patients identify. Classic complaints include numbness, coldness, cramping, and shooting pains. While "glove and stocking" distribution neuropathy is associated with this deficiency, most cases begin in the feet, and rarely are all limbs affected at once. Additionally, despite textbook teaching of bilateral symptoms, up to one-third of patients will report symptoms of neuropathy in one area only, such as a single foot. Associated complaints may include clumsiness and gait abnormality.

Depression and mild dementia are also reported as common symptoms of B12 deficiency.[7] Although these can actually be presenting symptoms, they may be difficult to distinguish as there are no features that would identify B12 as the cause.

Other complaints are typically manifestations of more advanced disease or are more rare. These may include (in no particular order) confusion, altered mental status, burning of the lip and mouth, ataxia, spasticity, contractures, paraplegia, muscular wasting, optic atrophy, delusions, disorientation, orthostatic hypotension, and psychosis.

**Laboratory evaluation.** *Serum B12.* Medical thinking regarding the correct method for evaluating B12 nutrition has changed significantly in the past decade. The most common screening method, serum B12, has come under much criticism, as it is now believed that this test may not identify many patients with clinically significant problems. Studies comparing serum B12 to other tests—homocysteine and methylmalonic acid (MMA)—have found that as few as 10 percent but perhaps as high as 50 percent of deficiencies may be missed by this test alone. Still, serum B12 is a cost-effective and simple screening test. Most US laboratories set the normal range for serum B12 at 200 to 900pg/mL. With current assays, very low levels (below 100) are almost 100-percent accurate in identifying deficiency. For levels between 100 and 400, this is not so clear-cut. Moreover, low folate status can cause a false low serum vitamin B12.[8] Thus, added tests for low-range patients will help identify deficiency.

For these reasons, and based on the high incidence of B12 deficiency after bariatric surgery, it is advisable that a comprehensive screen, including homocysteine and MMA, be performed in patients whose B12 levels are between 100pg/mL and 400pg/mL. This screening is the most accurate method for definitive diagnosis of B12 deficiency.

*Homocysteine.* In recent years, homocysteine has taken on new notoriety as an independent risk factor for cardiovascular disease. Additionally, elevations are linked to birth defects, arthritis, osteoporosis, dementia, and complications of diabetes.[9] Homocysteine is actually a byproduct of methionine metabolism that can build up when there is not enough B12 and/or folate for the methylation reaction that converts the homocysteine back to methionine. Some homocysteine can also undergo transsulfuration to cysteine via a B6-dependent reaction, but this is not considered a primary pathway of elimination. Homocysteine elevation is considered very sensitive for early B12 deficiency, but is not specific since it can also reflect folate and, to some degree, B6 deficiencies. Also worth noting is that increased protein intake may also cause a rise in homocysteine. Since higher protein intake is common in WLS patients, this could contribute to homocysteine elevation.

*Methylmalonic acid.* By contrast, levels of MMA are elevated only with B12 deficiency. MMA may be the very first functional sign of deficiency and will even detect subclinical deficiency. As mentioned above, when MMA and homocysteine are both elevated, a certain diagnosis of B12 deficiency can be made. If MMA is normal and homocysteine is elevated, other causes of elevated homocysteine should be explored.

*Hematologic manifestations.* Classically, B12 deficiency is associated with a macrocytic anemia (MCV >100), hypersegmented neutrophils, leucopenia, and thrombocytopenia. However, normocytic anemia can also occur; thus, macrocytosis is not a criteria. Also worth noting is that anemia of B12 deficiency only occurs after there has been enough depletion over enough time to decrease DNA synthesis, making it a relatively late sign. Routine chemistries may also show elevated bilirubin (indirect) and lactate dehydrogenase (LDH).

*Electrodiagnostic testing.* In those patients with B12 deficiency, electrodiagnostic abnormalities may be seen even in patients not reporting symptoms of neuropathy. Nerve conduction velocities tend to show decreased motor and/or sensory conduction and amplitude. Fibrillations and positive sharp waves may be present on electromyography. These tests can be useful in establishing severity of disease and monitoring recovery in patients with neuropathy or myelopathy. Additional changes can be seen in visual evoked potential (prolonged P100 wave) and somatosensory evoked potential (prolonged L3-P27 latency).

*Imaging.* Several magnetic resonance imaging (MRI) abnormalities have been reported in association with B12 deficiency. The most common appears to be increased T2-weighted signal in the posterior columns of the cervical thoracic cord. Fluid-attenuated inversion recovery (FLAIR) may show intensities in the posterior thoracic column and in the fourth ventricle of the brain. Swelling of the cervical and thoracic cord may be observed on T1 or T2 weighted imaging.

*Other tests.* Holotranscobalamin II is thought to be a very sensitive test for early depletion of vitamin B12. This test measures B12 bound to the primary carrier proteins in plasma— transcobalamin and haptocorrin. Because these proteins carry B12 to the cells, this test is considered to be a measurement of "usable" B12 in the body. Currently, this test has limited availability and is costly, but may one day become an excellent early screening method for B12 deficiency.

The Schilling test is an older test used to assess absorption of B12 due to lack of intrinsic factor or gastric acid.[10] This test was traditionally used in patients with pernicious anemia to see whether they could use oral B12 or required injections. The test is generally difficult to perform, and there are problems with interpretation. Moreover, it would be of specious use in gastric bypass patients who lack both of these factors anyway.

## PREVENTION AND TREATMENT

Vitamin B12 prophylaxis is simple and inexpensive and is clearly very important for patients who have undergone a malabsorptive procedure. Daily requirements of B12 are small, but the absorption when IF and gastric acid are low is greatly impaired. Studies indicate that large oral doses (greater than 500mcg) are well tolerated and well absorbed even in patients with pernicious anemia. A 2003 review article in *American Family Physician*[11] recommends daily dosing of 1000mcg. Alternately, an injection of 1000mcg per month is an accepted preventive dose. It is important that B12 injections be given intramuscularly. Clinicians administering the injections should be sure to use a long enough needle. If injecting into the gluteus medius, a 1.5-inch needle may be required depending on the amount of adipose tissue present. Vitamin B12 is very safe. To date, the Institute of

Medicine has not set a Tolerable Upper Limit for B12. Toxicity has never been demonstrated even at doses 10,000 times the RDA. Clinicians are sometimes alarmed by a high serum level of B12, but should understand that this is harmless and most likely reflects a recent dose of a dietary supplement or injection.

A diagnosis of B12 deficiency should be taken seriously and treated aggressively. If using oral or sublingual dosing, 2000mcg per day for 2 to 4 weeks is recommended. If injecting B12, 1000mcg daily for 1 to 2 weeks is usually adequate. These regimens should transition into the maintenance doses. Patients should be followed closely for clinical resolution. Anemia should begin to correct within the first two weeks. Comprehensive labs should be rechecked at 2 to 3 months. Repeat courses of therapy may be needed in some cases. Advanced neuropathies that do not begin to resolve in this period should be referred to a neurologist for consult or management. Some patients, unfortunately, can have permanent damage if treatment has been initiated too late.

While patients should be encouraged to include B12-rich foods in their diets, it is unlikely that patients with malabsorptive procedures will absorb much from dietary sources. B12-rich foods include meat, eggs, and dairy products.

## INTERACTIONS

B12 supplements can interfere with the absorption of some antibiotics (notably tetracycline). This is easily remedied by taking them two or more hours apart. Medications that lower gastric acid, including antacids, PPIs, and H2-blockers, can reduce B12 absorption. While this is likely insignificant in gastric bypass patients, it may minimize B12 absorption in other procedures. Some medications for diabetes and epilepsy can impair B12 status over time due to altered metabolism. Large doses of folate can correct the anemia of B12 deficiency, thus potentially masking it. If patients also have low iron stores, it should be noted that treatment of B12 deficiency may produce a further lowering of iron levels due to increased erythropoiesis. Thus, if trying to correct a combined deficiency, a temporary increase in iron supplementation may be required.

## CONCLUSION

B12 deficiency is a relatively common occurrence after WLS, increasing with patient age and the distance from the date of surgery. It is most common in RNY, but can occur with any procedure. Prevention is simple and inexpensive, especially in light of the potentially serious and permanent effects of B12 deficiency. Patients should be told about the effects of B12 deficiency and all attempts should be made to encourage adherence with prophylaxis. B12 labs should be part of regular screenings in WLS patients. The limitations of these screening tests must be recognized, and additional tests should be ordered to confirm or rule out deficiency as indicated. Finally, studies have shown that attending nutritional classes after WLS reduces overall incidence of neuropathy, including that caused by B12 deficiency.[12] Patients should be encouraged to attend postoperative support groups and classes to reduce their risk of B12 deficiency.

# REFERENCES

1.  Stramentinoli G. Pharmacologic aspects of S-adenosylmethionine: Pharmacokinetics and pharmacodynamics. *Am J Med* 1987;83(5A):35–42.
2.  Elia M. Oral or parenteral therapy for B12 deficiency. *Lancet* 1998;352:1721–2.
3.  Renshaw AA, Rabaza JR, Gonzalez AM, Verdeja JC. *Helicobacter pylori* infection in patients undergoing gastric bypass surgery for morbid obesity. *Obes Surg* 2001;11(3):281–3.
4.  Brolin RE, Leung M. Survey of vitamin and mineral supplementation after gastric bypass and biliopancreatic diversion for morbid obesity. *Obes Surg* 1999;9(2):150–4.
5.  Printen KJ, Halverson JD. Hemic micronutrients following vertical banded gastroplasty. *Am Surg* 1988;54(5):267–8.
6.  Dixon JB, Dixon ME, O'Brien PE. Elevated homocysteine levels with weight loss after Lap-Band surgery: Higher folate and vitamin B12 levels required to maintain homocysteine level. *Int J Obes Relat Metab Disord* 2001;25(2):219–27.
7.  Coppen A, Bolander-Gouaille C. Treatment of depression: Time to consider folic acid and vitamin B12. *J Psychopharmacol* 2005;19(1):59–65.
8.  Snow CF. Laboratory diagnosis of vitamin B12 and folate deficiency: A guide for the primary care physician. *Arch Intern Med* 1999;159:1289–98.
9.  Kuo HK, Sorond FA, Chen JH, et al. The role of homocysteine in multisystem age-related problems: A systematic review. *J Gerontol A Biol Sci Med Sci* 2005;60(9):1190–201.
10. Stabler SP. Screening the older population for cobalamin (vitamin B12) deficiency. *J Am Geriatr Soc* 1995;43:1290–7.
11. Oh R, Brown DL. Vitamin B12 deficiency. *Am Fam Physician* 2003;67(5):979–86.
12. Thaisetthawatkul P, Collazo-Clavell ML, Sarr MG, et al. A controlled study of peripheral neuropathy after bariatric surgery. *Neurology* 2004;63(8):1462–70.

# CHAPTER 6

# Vitamin A (Retinol)

Vitamin A is one of the four fat-soluble vitamins. The terms *vitamin A* and *pre-formed vitamin A* are used to refer to the retinoids—retinol, retinal, and retinoic acid. *Provitamin A* is a term that refers to certain red, orange, and yellow plant pigments called carotenoids. Of the 400 or more carotenoids found in nature, about 10 percent can be converted to vitamin A in the body. These carotenoids are called provitamin A, as they are considered to be a precursor source of retinoids. The most abundant and important provitamin A carotenoid is beta-carotene.

Retinoids and carotenoids in nature are usually protein bound. This means they must undergo hydrolysis in the stomach via pepsin. This process can also occur in the proximal small intestine via pancreatic enzymes. Some brush-border enzymes may also play a role in hydrolysis. After hydrolysis has occurred, these substances combine with other dietary fats into micelles, which can then be absorbed in the duodenum and jejunum via passive diffusion. Retinol absorption tends to be much more efficient than carotenoid absorption. In fact, it is estimated that 70 to 90 percent of retinol is absorbed while perhaps 20 to 50 percent of carotenoids are absorbed.[9] Absorption is also rapid, with the majority of uptake occurring within six hours of digestion. Uptake can occur throughout the duodenum and jejunum.

Once absorbed, most retinoids are carried to target cells or to the liver (for storage or excretion). Storage in the liver occurs along with some dietary fats in special cells called stellate cells. True hypervitaminosis A can only occur if the stellate cells have been overloaded with vitamin A. The liver can store nearly a year's supply of vitamin A, so deficiencies can take time to develop. Stored retinol can be mobilized whenever the body needs it. Retinol traveling in the body is carried by retinol-binding protein (RBP). The complex of RBP and retinol further binds to prealbumin (transthyretin or TTR). Carotenes can be stored in fat tissue anywhere in the body, and can be converted to vitamin A on an as-needed basis if body stores of retinol become low.

Vitamin A has numerous and diverse functions in human health. In the eyes, vitamin A is important for maintaining the health of the retina and transmitting light that comes into the eye into nerve signals. Retinal, formed from retinol through a zinc-dependent process, is particularly important to the function of rod cells. Rods transmit low light signals, accounting for much of a person's night vision. Because of this, one of the serious effects of vitamin A deficiency is night blindness. Normal immunity is vitamin-A dependent, and vitamin A is especially important to mucosal immunity in the lungs, sinuses, gastrointestinal system, urinary tract, and skin. Retinoids also assist in the differentiation of white blood cells and lymphocyte activation. Red blood cells (RBC) depend on vitamin A for differentiation as well. Furthermore, vitamin A plays a role in the transport of iron into the hemoglobin of developing RBCs. Some of the most critical physiologic actions of retinol are hormonal. In conjunction with vitamin D and thyroid hormone, the retinoic acid form of vitamin A works to both stimulate and inhibit some of the genes involved in cellular differentiation. In this way, growth and development are also vitamin-A dependent—both too much and too little vitamin A can cause defects of limbs, heart, eyes, and ears in fetal development. Regulation of growth hormone production is similarly dependent on vitamin A signaling. Retinoids and carotenoids also have the ability to act as antioxidants.

## DEFICIENCY

Vitamin A deficiency can result in serious health problems. The incidence of vitamin A deficiency after biliopancreatic diversion (BPD) and duodenal switch (DS) is estimated between 6 and 20 percent[1] and is undocumented after other procedures. Pathology of the eye is probably the best-recognized sign of retinol depletion. *Xerophthalmia* is the general term that describes manifestations of vitamin A deficiency in the eye. Patients with vitamin A deficiency may experience loss of night vision and extreme eye dryness. They may also report stumbling over things in the dark, a need to turn on lights earlier in the day, or difficulty driving after dusk. However, because of the abundance of electrical lighting, this symptom may go unnoticed. Clinicians may see Bitot's spots, keratomalacia, poor dark adaptation, or corneal ulcers. Patients

| 1 retinol equivalent (RE) | = 1mcg retinol |
|---|---|
| | = 6mcg beta carotene |
| | = 12mcg other carotenoids |
| 1IU (international unit) | = 0.3mcg retinol |
| 1mcg retinol | = 3.3IU |

with vitamin A deficiency may also suffer from low tear production. Fundoscopic examination may show small pale spots in the retina. Severe vitamin A deficiency can cause total blindness.

Those with vitamin A deficiency may have problems with skin and mucous membranes due to keratin accumulation. These can include dry skin, dry hair, broken nails, follicular hyperkeratosis (especially of the arms and thighs), itching, and generally rough or bumpy skin. Increased incidence of infection (especially of the respiratory, genitourinary, and gastrointestinal systems) and poor wound healing are signs of impaired vitamin A-mediated immunity. Additionally, low sperm counts in men (impaired spermatogenesis) and history of spontaneous abortion in women can be signs of a subclinical deficiency. Vitamin A deficiency can also cause increased deposition of periosteal bone and possible increased incidence of kidney stone formation.

Deficiency of vitamin A with malabsorptive procedures is likely to be most directly related to the length of the intestine that has been bypassed. The more fat malabsorption that occurs, the more vitamin A malabsorption. The need for retinoids from food to undergo hydrolysis in the stomach may also contribute to deficiency. Secondary axes of deficiency are related to the dependency of vitamin A on other aspects of nutrition. For example, protein and zinc are both required for RBP; thus, low intake or deficiency of either could cause or exacerbate a vitamin A deficiency. Low-calorie intake is also a cause of vitamin A deficiency. Furthermore, vitamin A and iron are interdependent on each other.[2] Many studies have shown that resistant iron deficiency corrects more easily with concurrent vitamin A supplementation. A smaller number of studies indicate that vitamin A deficiency can contribute to the development of iron deficiency due to the role that retinol plays in the transport of iron into hemoglobin in RBC formation. As with many nutrients, excessive alcohol consumption is also a risk for deficiency, as is chronic diarrhea.

## LABORATORY EVALUATION

Serum or plasma levels of retinol are an inexpensive and accurate assessment of vitamin A nutrition, reflecting both liver storage and dietary intake. Levels of less than 1.05μmol/L (20μg/dL) are considered in the deficient range by most standards. If low vitamin A is found on a screening test in a weight loss surgery (WLS) patient, other tests are recommended. RBP should be screened, as a protein deficiency could result in low circulating retinol with ample liver stores. For the same reason, zinc status should be assessed as well. Prealbumin and albumin can also be measured as additional assessments for protein nutrition. Assessing iron status and anemia is also a good idea as the deficiencies often coexist.

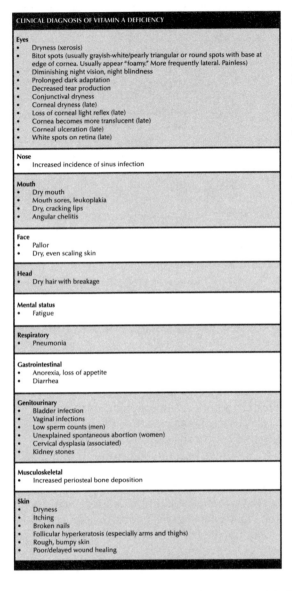

**CLINICAL DIAGNOSIS OF VITAMIN A DEFICIENCY**

**Eyes**
- Dryness (xerosis)
- Bitot spots (usually grayish-white/pearly triangular or round spots with base at edge of cornea. Usually appear "foamy." More frequently lateral. Painless)
- Diminishing night vision, night blindness
- Prolonged dark adaptation
- Decreased tear production
- Conjunctival dryness
- Corneal dryness (late)
- Loss of corneal light reflex (late)
- Cornea becomes more translucent (late)
- Corneal ulceration (late)
- White spots on retina (late)

**Nose**
- Increased incidence of sinus infection

**Mouth**
- Dry mouth
- Mouth sores, leukoplakia
- Dry, cracking lips
- Angular chelitis

**Face**
- Pallor
- Dry, even scaling skin

**Head**
- Dry hair with breakage

**Mental status**
- Fatigue

**Respiratory**
- Pneumonia

**Gastrointestinal**
- Anorexia, loss of appetite
- Diarrhea

**Genitourinary**
- Bladder infection
- Vaginal infections
- Low sperm counts (men)
- Unexplained spontaneous abortion (women)
- Cervical dysplasia (associated)
- Kidney stones

**Musculoskeletal**
- Increased periosteal bone deposition

**Skin**
- Dryness
- Itching
- Broken nails
- Follicular hyperkeratosis (especially arms and thighs)
- Rough, bumpy skin
- Poor/delayed wound healing

Since the liver holds more than 90 percent of the body stores of vitamin A, liver biopsy has been used to establish reserves. However, since serum levels of retinol have been shown to correlate well with liver stores in the absence of protein and zinc deficiency, liver biopsy should be an unnecessary, invasive procedure. Conjunctival cytology has been used as a screening test in many third-world nations, but has not demonstrated accuracy in finding early deficiency.

In the presence of eye disease, clinical assessment correlates accurately to the degree of vitamin A deficiency. A history of night blindness, in particular, has been found to be a fairly specific screening tool in children in areas where vitamin A deficiency is endemic. The Dark Adaptation Test is an early measure of vitamin A nutrition, even detecting subclinical deficiency; however, it is considered too time-consuming to be clinically practical. The test takes about 45 minutes to perform in the office and requires a dedicated, light-proof room. An electroretinogram is generally performed by an ophthalmologist and may be useful in distinguishing retinal problems due to vitamin A deficiency from those due to other causes. This test might be useful to assess a patient who appears to have retinol deficiency, but also has a history of a condition such as diabetic retinopathy.

Carotenoids can be assessed individually in plasma or serum. There is no recommended daily allowance (RDA) for carotenoids and no documented deficiency with WLS. However, for interested clinicians, measurements are available for many carotenoids, including beta-carotene, alpha-carotene, lycopene, lutein, and zeaxanthin. These assays are heavily influenced by dietary intakes.

## TREATMENT

Treatment of vitamin A deficiency may vary depending on whether there is eye involvement. In the absence of xerophthalmia, a good initial treatment is a dose of 100,000IU of retinol as an

| PLASMA RETINOL | |
|---|---|
| ≥30mcg/100mL | Normal |
| 30–20mcg/100mL | Mild deficiency, associated with night blindness, Bitot's spots |
| 20–10mcg/100mL | Moderate deficiency |
| <10mcg/100mL | Definitely low, severe deficiency |

oral preparation or intramuscularly (IM) for three days, followed by 50,000IU for two weeks. Maintaining a daily level of 20,000IU for 2 to 3 months is then advisable. Xerophthalmia should be treated as a medical emergency because of the serious risk of blindness. Progression to corneal involvement is generally irreversible. If any degree of xerophthalmia is present, intramuscular injection of 200,000IU should be administered immediately. The same dose can be repeated in 24 hours, then again in two weeks. It has alternately been suggested that 500,000IU orally for three days be given. Either of these regimens can be followed by 50,000IU for two weeks and then 20,000IU for several months.

Both oral and IM vitamin A are available in several types of preparations. When treating a true deficiency, it is important to use preformed vitamin A and not beta-carotene. The most common IM preparation used is water-miscible vitamin A palmitate. Oral preparations can be found both in oil-based soft gels (often blended with vitamin D) or as water-miscible forms. The latter are better absorbed,[3] making them preferable; however, they can also produce toxicity more easily.[4] Common preparations of vitamin A are retinyl palmitate or retinyl acetate. Common doses include 5,000, 8,000, 10,000, and 25,000IU.

High-dose vitamin A treatment must be closely monitored as significant side effects can result. Acute toxicity can occur within hours to a few days of a large bolus dose. Symptoms may include nausea, vomiting, blurred vision, headache, and vertigo. Symptoms will usually resolve rapidly, within 1 to 2 days. Peeling skin, hair loss, and bone pain may develop a few days later. Chronic toxicity can produce a range of symptoms including hair loss, anorexia, bone pain, liver and spleen enlargement, cheilitis, rashes/peeling, pseudotumor cerebri, and hyperpigmentation. Osteoporosis is also a risk of chronic vitamin A overload.

Due to the known teratogenic nature of retinol, great caution should be taken in pregnancy or possible pregnancy. Non-pregnant women who are on high-dose vitamin A therapy should be warned of the potential harm to a fetus as a result of taking daily levels of more than 10,000IU per day. However, clinicians should note that the risk of doses between 10,000 and 30,000IU appears small.[5] In women with malabsorptive procedures who are planning a pregnancy, it would be best to determine vitamin A levels preconceptually and treat any problems in advance. A vitamin A-deficient woman who becomes pregnant presents a challenging clinical situation, as both low and high vitamin A can harm fetal development. Clinical decision making in a case such as this should involve a multidisciplinary team, including members of the bariatric team as well as a high-risk obstetric specialist.

| XEROPHTHALMIA -PROGRESSION AND GRADING (WHO) |
|:---:|
| **REVERSIBLE CHANGES** |
| **XN Night blindness** |
| **XIA Conjunctival xerosis** |
| **XIB With Bitot's spot** |
| **IRREVERSIBLE CHANGES** |
| **X2 Corneal xerosis** |
| **X3A Corneal Ulceration (<1/3)** |
| **X3B Keratomalcia (>1/3)** |
| **XS Corneal scar from xerophthalmia** |

## PREVENTION AND MAINTENANCE

The exact amount of vitamin A required to prevent deficiency after Roux-en-y (RNY) or DS surgeries is unknown. The RDA for vitamin A is 3,000IU (900mcg). The tolerable upper limit (UL) is set at 10,000IU (3000mcg). However, chronic ingestion of over 5,000IU per day is associated with increased risk of osteoporosis in individuals without malabsorption.[6] There is no upper limit for beta-carotene, as toxicity has not been observed even at very high doses over long periods of time. Daily doses of 10,000 to 20,000IU of retinol are not uncommon for prevention in programs performing DS procedures. Lower doses, in the range of 5,000 to 10,000IU, are more common with RNY. Multivitamin preparations containing up to 10,000IU are readily available in many forms. A separate vitamin A product may be required to reach higher daily doses. Because there have been cases of permanent blindness caused by vitamin A deficiency,[7] patients with significant malabsorption should be educated about the importance of adhering to prescribed supplements and reporting for regular lab work.

Preformed vitamin A is not common in foods other than liver, fortified milk, egg yolk, and fortified breakfast cereals. Beta-carotene and other carotenoids are found throughout the plant world in colorful fruits and vegetables. Although it is important for general health that patients include these foods in their diets, patients with malabsorption cannot fully depend on these foods for maintaining vitamin A levels in the body.

## INTERACTIONS

Numerous drugs interact with retinol. Oral contraceptives and statins can increase serum levels of vitamin A with long-term use. Isotretinoin, a synthetic derivative of vitamin A (Accutane®), should not be taken with retinol without close physician supervision. Caution should also be used with topical retinoids. Medroxyprogesterone, methyltestosterone, oral corticosteroids, bile acid sequestrants, orlistat, and some anticonvulsants and antibiotic classes can all lower vitamin A levels. Patients taking these drugs who are also at risk for vitamin A deficiency may require closer monitoring.

Other nutrients also interact with vitamin A. Both transport and use of vitamin A require adequate protein status. Therefore, low protein can contribute to vitamin A deficiency. Vitamin A interacts with the other three fat-soluble vitamins in different ways. Low vitamin E can decrease the conversion of beta-carotene to retinol, and high intake of vitamin A can reduce absorption of vitamin K and interfere with vitamin D-dependent calcium uptake.[8] As stated above, these interferences with vitamin D activity has led to some rethinking about recommended levels of preformed retinol. The conversion of retinol in the body to retinal is dependent on zinc. Since the formation of retinal from retinol requires zinc, low zinc status can alter night vision and visual acuity without signs of xerophthalmia. Low vitamin A can also contribute to iron deficiency anemia as discussed in the section on absorption. Finally, regular alcohol intake increases the potential toxicity of vitamin A. Patients taking high-dose vitamin A should be advised to avoid alcohol intake.

## CONCLUSION

Vitamin A deficiency carries serious risks. Patients who have undergone malabsorptive procedures for weight loss should be monitored regularly and educated in prevention, including warning signs of deficiency. Incidence of vitamin A deficiency in RNY is unknown because it is typically not assessed, but this does not mean that it does not occur. Although there is not enough data to recommend regular screening of retinol levels in all RNY patients, clinicians need to be aware that vitamin A deficiency can occur. Being familiar with early clinical presentation will help healthcare professionals understand when they do need to screen. Asking simple questions about vision, night driving, and skin problems can help identify at-risk patients. Additionally, patients with resistant iron deficiency should be screened for vitamin A deficiency since this may be a hidden cause.

## REFERENCES

1. Brolin RE, Leung M. Survey of vitamin and mineral supplementation after gastric bypass and biliopancreatic diversion for morbid obesity. *Obes Surg* 1999;9(2):150–4.
2. Karyadi D, Bloem MW. The role of vitamin A in iron deficiency anemia and implications for interventions. *Biomedical and Environmental Sciences* 1996;9:316–24.
3. Lewis J, Bodansky O, Birmingham J, Cohlan S. Vitamin A. Comparative absorption, excretion and storage of oily and aqueous preparations. *J Pediatr* 1947;31:496–508.
4. Myhre AM, Carlsen MH, Bohn SK, et al. Water-miscible, emulsified, and solid forms of retinol supplements are more toxic than oil-based preparations. *Am J Clin Nutr* 2003;78(6):1152–9.
5. Miller RK, Hendrickx AG, Mills JL, et al. Periconceptional vitamin A use: How much is teratogenic? *Reprod Toxicol* 1998;12(1):75–88.
6. Michaelsson K, Lithell H, Vessby B, Melhus H. Serum retinol levels and the risk of fracture. *N Engl J Med* 2003;348(4):287–94.
7. Scopinaro N, Gianetta E, Adami GF, et al. Biliopancreatic diversion for obesity at eighteen years. *Surgery* 1996;119:261–8.
8. Johansson S, Melhus H. Vitamin A antagonizes calcium response to vitamin D in man. *J Bone Miner Res* 2001;16(10):1899–1905.
9. Food and Nutrition Board, Institute of Medicine. *Dietary Reference Intakes for Vitamin A, Vitamin K, Arsenic, Boron, Chromium, Copper, Iodine, Iron, Manganese, Molybdenum, Nickel, Silicon, Vanadium, and Zinc.* Washington, DC: National Academies Press, 2000.

# CHAPTER 7

# Vitamin D

Vitamin D is one of the fat-soluble vitamins and is also a steroid hormone. Some scientists have, in fact, argued that vitamin D should not be classified as a vitamin at all. Typically, the definition of a vitamin is an organic substance that is necessary for human health and cannot be manufactured by the body. Vitamin D, however, is manufactured in skin from a reaction with ultraviolet light. In theory, humans should not require dietary sources unless we lack adequate sunlight. However, not all theories translate well to reality. There appears to be a conditional need for exogenous vitamin D for many people. Therefore, the dual classification is what is currently best accepted.

On paper, vitamin D's chemical structure looks very much like any other steroid hormone the body makes, such as estrogen, progesterone, testosterone, and cortisol. Precursors to active vitamin D are found both in the human body and in irradiated foods. To be utilized, these precursors must go through a series of complex transformations that involve the skin, liver, and kidneys. We did not really understand much about the process until it was studied in the 1970s, and even now, we are still uncovering new complexities to how vitamin D and its related hormones work.

There are seven identified forms of vitamin D, of which two forms are most commonly known: D2 (ergocalciferol) and D3 (cholecalciferol). The most familiar form is D2, which is also the most common commercial form because it can be readily prepared from plant materials that contain the compound ergosterol. Vitamin D3 is the form that animals (including humans) synthesize from cholesterol. This happens when a form of cholesterol (7-dehydro) travels to the skin and interacts with ultraviolet light. D3 and its active metabolites, 25-hydroxy and 1,25-dihydroxycholecalciferol, are considered to be the most potent forms.[1]

Being fatty in nature, dietary forms of vitamin D are absorbed together with fats from food. This primarily happens in the jejunum and ileum. Absorption also depends on interaction with bile salts that come from the liver. Any condition that results in a diminished ability to absorb fat will result in a diminished ability to absorb vitamin D. This can include a condition like Crohn's disease or weight loss surgeries, such as gastric bypass (GB) or duodenal switch (DS).

Absorption in the intestines ultimately occurs by the slow process of passive diffusion. After absorption occurs, vitamin D is transported by its own binding protein (vitamin D binding protein, DBP) to tissues where it is metabolized or utilized. It is worth noting that DBP is dependent on vitamin D for its synthesis—thus in deficiency states, there may be a complicating factor of diminished DBP to carry the available hormone.[2]

As with all steroid hormones, the synthesis of vitamin D begins with cholesterol. 7-dehydrocholesterol travels to the surface of the skin where, in the presence of adequate sunlight, it is converted to cholecalciferol (D3). Cholecalciferol, in turn, is metabolized first in the liver to 25-hydroxycholecalciferol, then in the kidneys to the active hormone 1,25-dihydroxycholecalciferol. Under ideal circumstances, this mechanism should supply enough vitamin D such that dietary and supplemental forms are not needed in the presence of adequate sunlight exposure. It is estimated that in the summer, 15 minutes three times a week of exposing the hands, arms, and face (without sunscreen) to early morning or late afternoon sun will make all the vitamin D one needs. Dark skinned individuals require 5 to 10 times this exposure. For reasons discussed later, however, this production mechanism may not be adequate for some people.

The body also recycles vitamin D from bile (the major route of excretion for D and other steroids). This mechanism is believed to act as a back-up system to protect the body during times where sources from diet or sunlight may be unavailable. This may be another disadvantage for DS patients because in these patients, bile is dumped into the lower part of the small intestines only, providing little opportunity for this recycling to occur.[3]

Vitamin D plays numerous important roles in human health. Most actions of vitamin D are mediated through the vitamin D receptor or VDR. The VDR is a gene transcription protein found in cells that use vitamin D. The VDR is closely associated to the vitamin A receptor, and together the two regulate the expression of more than 50 genes in the human body. Thus, the impact of vitamin D on human health is far-reaching, with new functions regularly being discovered.

Best known is vitamin D's importance to the health of bone. 1,25-dihydroxy-D3 stimulates the production of a protein in the digestive system called calbindin. Calbindin allows the body to absorb calcium from the digestive system into the blood stream. Additionally, vitamin D acts upon the digestive system directly to make it more permeable to calcium. Vitamin D further regulates blood calcium levels, being able to both increase and decrease levels based on demand. Vitamin D is also critical to the ability of the body to deposit calcium in bone. This is part of a complex interaction between 1,25-dihydroxy-D3 and parathyroid hormone. When both hormones are present in adequate levels, they work together to stimulate bone synthesis, but when D is low, the relative excess of parathyroid hormone stimulates a pathway by which more bone is broken down and lost. It is important to note that because of the interrelationship of vitamin D and calcium, low vitamin D can create the symptoms of low calcium. Additionally, active vitamin D is required for the synthesis of osteocalcin, a vitamin K-dependent bone protein.[4]

There has been particular attention paid lately to the role that vitamin D may play in immunity, specifically with respect to cancer. Numerous cancers, including breast, colon, prostate, bone, and melanoma, have been found to contain vitamin D receptors. We know that some active vitamin D analogs play a role in cell differentiation, and in some of these cancers we have evidence that vitamin D may be able to inhibit cancer cell proliferation and induce more normal cell synthesis. The strongest scientific evidence correlating low vitamin D status with cancer is with breast, prostate, and colon, and there is research looking at the potential for vitamin D's therapeutic potential in this area. Active vitamin D has also been found to have regulatory function in other parts of the immune system. There is emerging animal research that indicates that vitamin D status may play a role preventing some autoimmune diseases, such as multiple sclerosis, lupus, and rheumatoid arthritis.[5-8]

There is good research that vitamin D deficiency plays a role in the development of diabetes. We know that insulin release is impaired in the absence of adequate vitamin D. This is because insulin release is calcium dependent. This same mechanism may explain the correlation between polycystic ovarian syndrome and vitamin D. Vitamin D also has roles in some areas of fetal and placental development, deoxyribonucleic acid (DNA) transcription, pituitary function, and possibly heart health. With growing research on many of these aspects of vitamin D, we are likely to learn a great deal more in the coming decades about the roles it plays in human health.[5-8]

## DEFICIENCY

Vitamin D status can become impaired for several reasons, including decreased exposure to sunlight (see sidebar), low dietary intake, age, skin color, and malabsorption. Kidney or liver disease can also contribute to deficiency if the ability to synthesize vitamin D is impaired. Vitamin D deficiency has been reported in both pre- and postoperative weight loss surgery patients. As discussed in Chapter 1, preoperative rates of deficiency in weight loss surgery (WLS) patients may be as high as 62 percent.[9] Following duodenal switch (DS) and Roux-en-y gastric bypass (RNY), there is increased risk due to fat malabsorption, which will include to varying degrees loss of fat-soluble vitamins. Vitamin D deficiency can occur in 50 percent or

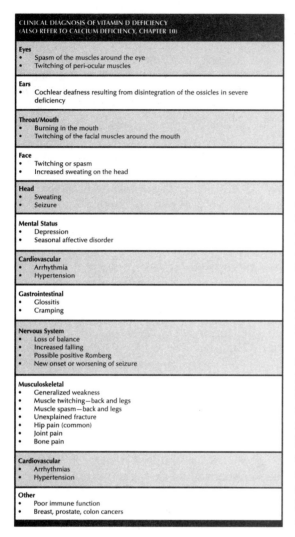

| CLINICAL DIAGNOSIS OF VITAMIN D DEFICIENCY (ALSO REFER TO CALCIUM DEFICIENCY, CHAPTER 10) |
| --- |
| **Eyes** |
| • Spasm of the muscles around the eye |
| • Twitching of peri-ocular muscles |
| **Ears** |
| • Cochlear deafness resulting from disintegration of the ossicles in severe deficiency |
| **Throat/Mouth** |
| • Burning in the mouth |
| • Twitching of the facial muscles around the mouth |
| **Face** |
| • Twitching or spasm |
| • Increased sweating on the head |
| **Head** |
| • Sweating |
| • Seizure |
| **Mental Status** |
| • Depression |
| • Seasonal affective disorder |
| **Cardiovascular** |
| • Arrhythmia |
| • Hypertension |
| **Gastrointestinal** |
| • Glossitis |
| • Cramping |
| **Nervous System** |
| • Loss of balance |
| • Increased falling |
| • Possible positive Romberg |
| • New onset or worsening of seizure |
| **Musculoskeletal** |
| • Generalized weakness |
| • Muscle twitching—back and legs |
| • Muscle spasm—back and legs |
| • Unexplained fracture |
| • Hip pain (common) |
| • Joint pain |
| • Bone pain |
| **Cardiovascular** |
| • Arrhythmias |
| • Hypertension |
| **Other** |
| • Poor immune function |
| • Breast, prostate, colon cancers |

more of DS patients[10] and is one of the more serious risks. At least one study has reported vitamin D deficiency as one of the most common deficiency states with RNY;[11] however, as most programs do not routinely screen for vitamin D, the true incidence is unknown. Vitamin D status appears to remain stable with adjustable gastric banding (AGB), despite other evidence for negative bone remodeling.[12]

For the most part, vitamin D deficiency is a silent condition. Bone loss, evidenced on imaging studies as osteomalacia and osteoporosis, is usually the first finding. Most, if any, physical signs are related to subsequent calcium deficiency (see Chapter 10 for complete signs and symptoms of calcium deficiency). This syndrome is called rachitic tetany. These symptoms include muscle pain and weakness, muscle spasm (especially in the back and legs), facial spasms, muscle twitching, unexplained fracture, joint pain (especially hip pain), bone pain, and possible hearing loss (due to the ear ossicles dissolving). Other possible features include increased head sweating, burning in the mouth, increased incidence of dysmenorrhea in women, seasonal affective disorder (SAD), cardiac arrhythmias, seizures, fatigue, loss of balance/falling, hypertension, and poor immune function (including cancer).

# DIAGNOSIS

Because of the silent, subclinical nature of vitamin D deficiency, laboratory diagnosis is important in establishing patient status. The most accurate tests for vitamin D deficiency are serum 25-hydroxycholecalciferol. This is also called 25-hydroxy-vitamin D and 25(OH)D. There has been debate in recent years as to the accuracy of the reference ranges for 25 (OH)D since there is so much variation based on age, skin tone, and geographic location that do not correlate with health status. The current thinking in the laboratory community is that a more accurate assessment is provided by correlating vitamin D levels with parathormone (PTH) levels, giving a more complete picture of when the body responds to tissue deficiency. PTH will rise when vitamin D is deficient. When testing for PTH, it is best to use the measurement of

## SUN, SKIN, AND VITAMIN D

Inadequate exposure to the sun is a significant contributor to vitamin D deficiency. People who spend most of their daylight hours indoors, those who cover up for religious reasons, and those who, due to work or infirmity, do not get outside regularly during daylight hours are all at risk. Sunscreen also blocks the ultraviolet B rays from the sun that are required for vitamin D production. Sunscreens with an SPF of 8 and above block virtually all vitamin D synthesis. Where you live can also have an impact. In many areas of North America, above 40° latitude, there are inadequate levels of ultraviolet B rays available from November to March to assure vitamin D synthesis from sun exposure. In areas of Canada, this season may extend even further—October to April. Some studies have indicated that even in those who take a multivitamin containing vitamin D together with drinking milk, up to 80 percent of those individuals living in northern latitudes may be vitamin D deficient by the end of winter. Finally, the skin itself can have an impact. Darker skinned individuals, which is essentially like having a built-in SPF, require much greater UV exposure to produce the required amount of vitamin D. This is a particular problem for dark-skinned individuals of Indian or African descent who are living in northern latitudes. Moreover, the elderly have diminished production of vitamin D in the skin, which may be due to the thinning of skin with age.

1.    Holick MF. Vitamin D: Importance in the prevention of cancers, type 1 diabetes, heart disease, and osteoporosis. *Am J Clin Nutr* 2004;79(3):362–71.

intact PTH (iPTH), which looks at biologically active hormone only. Thus newer thinking suggests that true hypovitaminosis D occurs when vitamin D levels reach a point that PTH becomes slightly elevated. While many labs will define a low 25(OH)D as below 20ng/mL (50nmol/L), PTH levels may rise sooner, at levels of 30 to 40ng/mL. Since both tests are readily available, the combined assessment is advisable.

## OTHER LABS

Serum alkaline phosphatase is increased in osteomalacia and is usually normal with osteoporosis, but can also be altered for other reasons (such as advanced age and pregnancy). Intact osteocalcin (OC) levels are vitamin D-dependent and are known to rise in osteomalacia. Serum undercarboxylated osteocalcin (unOC) levels will rise with vitamin D deficiency, but also in response to other influences, such as vitamin K deficiency.[13] Levels of both OC and unOC may eventually prove to be useful in monitoring response to vitamin D therapy, but there is not enough evidence at this time to be certain. Very low levels of vitamin D (below 8ng/mL) are associated with serum hypocalcemia and hypophosphatemia. Urinary calcium levels will also fall.

Imaging studies can be useful in the assessment of vitamin D. X-ray may show diffuse osteopenia and pseudofractures ("Looser's Zones"). Since vitamin D has greater influence on cortical bone (legs, arms, hips) than on trabecular bone (spine, ribs, pelvis), greater or exclusive loss of bone at the hip relative to the spine, should indicate to the clinician the need to evaluate vitamin D status. Conversely, since there is a strong correlation between vitamin D deficiency and hip fracture, patients with low vitamin D and vitamin D malabsorption should have regular evaluations for bone density that include evaluation of the hip.

## TREATMENT

For low vitamin D, weekly dosing of 50,000IU as a dry, water-miscible form (versus in an oil filled soft gel) is a typical treatment. If levels are very low (at or below 8ng/mL with hypocalcemia), 50,000IU can be given daily for up to three weeks. This should be done under close supervision and monitoring for toxicity. In some cases, it may be necessary to use injectable preparations. Injection therapy requires closer monitoring of serum calcium, PTH, 25(OH)D, and alkaline phosphatase and should be administered by a professional experienced in managing this treatment. These more extreme deficiencies typically require calcium therapy as well, which may need to be intravenous. This is very important if there is acute, symptomatic hypocalcemia. For less severe deficiency, oral dosing with 50,000IU once weekly for 6 to 8 weeks is typical. Again, weekly injections of 50,000IU can also be considered. Alternately, 2000 to 5000IU per day can be considered. A final consideration would be a compounded transdermal preparation. Preparations with levels ranging from 600IU/gram to as high as 10,000IU/gram can be ordered. Creams or gels must be applied on areas where skin is thin, such as the inner wrist, to avoid vitamin D being taken up by adipose tissue. When body stores have been repleted (vitamin D levels above 30 with normalized PTH), then a maintenance dose can be implemented. Finally, it is very important that patients taking therapeutic doses of vitamin D take 1000 to 1500mg (or sometimes more) of calcium per day.

## PREVENTION AND MAINTENANCE

The question of what the correct maintenance dose of vitamin D is has not been answered. The adequate intake (AI) for adults is 200IU for ages 19 to 50; 400IU for ages 51 to 70; and 600 IU for ages 71 and older. These levels were last set in 1997 and are felt by many experts to be too low. The tolerable upper limit (UL) from all combined sources (diet and supplements) as set by the Institute of Medicine is 2000IU, but this is also debated. One thing that everyone agrees on is that a person cannot overdose on vitamin D from sunshine. Advising sun exposure at suberythemal doses can be beneficial for vitamin D status. This can be combined with a recommendation for exercise. Sun lamps and tanning beds are another alternative.

For patients who have undergone RNY, it is unknown whether doses of vitamin D greater than the AI are needed to maintain normal status; there is too little data. Since vitamin D levels are sensitive to many factors from geographic location to skin color, regular screening is the only way to know whether the level of vitamin D in an individual patient is being adequately maintained. Since there is a reasonable window of safety between the AI and the UL, clinicians can feel comfortable recommending higher maintenance doses. A good dose to consider is 800IU, which has reasonable support for prevention of vitamin D deficiency.[14] Doses above the AI should be considered in older adults, dark-skinned individuals, those who spend limited time outdoors, and those who are intolerant of dairy products.

With patients who have had DS, there is clearly a higher need for vitamin D nutrition. Even daily doses of 1200IU have still resulted in relatively high rates of deficiency.[15] While the UL is set at 2000IU, there is good evidence that levels up to 10,000IU per day are unlikely to produce toxicity in adults.[16] Therefore, as long as there is consistent follow-up, clinicians can feel comfortable recommending levels above the AI for DS patients.

## EXCESS/TOXICITY

Toxicity from vitamin D is a risk from supplemental sources and should be monitored in individuals who supplement at very high levels. The upper limit from all combined sources (diet and supplements) as set by the Institute of Medicine is 2000IU. As we have already noted, however, toxicity is unlikely even at 4 to 5 times that dose. Acute toxicity can produce anorexia, nausea, vomiting, itching, thirst, frequent urination, and agitation. There can also be renal impairment. Clinical signs of chronic excess may also include dizziness, fatigue, muscle cramping (which can be severe), muscle pain, muscle twitching, neuritis or neuropathy, and kidney stones. There is also a weak connection with excessive vitamin D intake and the presence of Bell's Palsy.

## INTERACTIONS

Vitamin D may interfere with the efficacy of verapamil, a type of calcium channel blocker medication. A single report in 1975 suggested that vitamin D might be a problem for people taking anticoagulants; however, no data since then has supported this thinking. The use of estrogen replacement may increase blood levels of vitamin D, although this has largely been viewed as a benefit and not a risk for toxicity. Some drugs interfere with absorption, metabolism, or utilization of vitamin D: Cimetidine interferes with the liver's role in activating vitamin D; long-term use of anticonvulsants is known to disrupt bone metabolism, and vitamin D has been shown to assist in the prevention of bone loss in these cases; both orlistat (a lipase inhibitor used for weight loss) and bile acid sequesterants inhibit the absorption of vitamin D; corticosteroids interfere with the activation and metabolism of vitamin D; and sunscreens block the ability of the body to synthesize vitamin D in the skin. Other interactions may apply as well; thus, it is a good idea for individuals who are vitamin D deficient to check with their pharmacist regarding possible interactions with their prescriptions.

## CONCLUSION

Vitamin D is clearly a complex nutrient playing many roles in long-term health and well-being. Clinicians should both understand the importance of getting enough vitamin D from sun, food, and supplements, as well as respect the problems that can arise from both deficiency and excess. When we look at the long-term health and wellness of WLS patients, I always think of vitamin D as a great example. While the weight loss that can result from the surgery can provide enormous health benefits, these benefits are not good trade-offs for a broken hip (causing serious disability or death) or cancer. Good nutritional counseling, lifestyle counseling, and regular lab work should help to reduce incidence of deficiency and catch the deficiencies that do occur at an earlier point.

# REFERENCES

1.  Brody T. *Nutritional Biochemistry, Second Edition.* San Diego, CA: Academic Press, 1999.
2.  Berdanier CE. *Advanced Micronutrition: Micronutrients.* Boca Raton, FL: CRC Press, 1998.
3.  DeLuca HF, Zierold C. Mechanisms and functions of vitamin D. *Nutr Rev* 1998;56(2 Pt 2):S4–10.
4.  Garland CF, Garland FC, Gorham ED. Calcium and vitamin D: Their potential roles in colon and breast cancer prevention. *Ann N Y Acad Sci* 1999;889:107–19.
5.  Food and Nutrition Board, Institute of Medicine. *Vitamin D. Dietary Reference Intakes: Calcium, Phosphorus, Magnesium, Vitamin D, and Fluoride.* Washington, DC: National Academy Press, 1997:250–87.
6.  Martinez ME, Giovannucci EL, Colditz GA, et al. Calcium, vitamin D, and the occurrence of colorectal cancer among women. *J Natl Cancer Inst* 1996;88(19):1375–82.
7.  Jahnsen J, Falch JA, Mowinckel P, Aadland E. Vitamin D status, parathyroid hormone and bone mineral density in patients with inflammatory bowel disease. *Scand J Gastroenterol* 2002;37(2):192–9.
8.  Shapses SA, Von Thun NL, Heymsfield SB, et al. Bone turnover and density in obese premenopausal women during moderate weight loss and calcium supplementation. *J Bone Miner Res* 2001 Jul;16(7):1329–36.
9.  Buffington C, Walker B, Cowan GS Jr, Scruggs D. Vitamin D deficiency in the morbidly obese. *Obes Surg* 1993;3(4):421–4.
10. Newbury L, Dolan K, Hatzifotis M, et al. Calcium and vitamin D depletion and elevated parathyroid hormone following biliopancreatic diversion. *Obes Surg* 2003;13(6):893–5.
11. Alvarez-Leite JI. Nutrient deficiencies secondary to bariatric surgery. *Curr Opin Clin Nutr Metab Care* 2004;7(5):569–75.
12. Pugnale N, Giusti V, Suter M, et al. Bone metabolism and risk of secondary hyperparathyroidism 12 months after gastric banding in obese pre-menopausal women. *Int J Obes Relat Metab Disord* 2003;27(1):110–6.
13. Szulc P Chapuy MC, Meunier PJ, Delmas PD. Serum undercarboxylated osteocalcin is a marker of the risk of hip fracture in elderly women. *J Clin Invest* 1993;91(4):1769–74.
14. Deitel M, Cowan GSM. *Update: Surgery for the Morbidly Obese Patient.* Philadelphia, PA: Lippincott, Williams, and Wilken, 2000.
15. Slater GH, Ren CJ, Siegel N, et al. Serum fat-soluble vitamin deficiency and abnormal calcium metabolism after malabsorptive bariatric surgery. *J Gastrointest Surg* 2004;8:48–55.
16. Vieth R. Vitamin D supplementation, 25-hydroxyvitamin D concentrations, and safety. *Am J Clin Nutr* 1999;69(5):842–56.

# CHAPTER 8

# Vitamin K

Vitamin K is a fat-soluble nutrient that is best known for its role in blood clotting. The term *vitamin K* actually applies to a group of chemicals with vitamin K activity. The three primary vitamin K compounds are K1 or phylloquinone (from plants), K2 or menaquinone (synthesized by intestinal flora), and K or menadione (a synthetic analog). There is also menatetrenone, a form of vitamin K2 that has garnered recent interest for treatment of bone loss.

Vitamin K1 is readily found in vegetables (especially leafy greens) and in vegetable oils. Fruits, meats, and grains also contain small amounts. Vitamin K2 is made in the large intestine by bacterial synthesis.

K1 is absorbed by an active transport mechanism in the jejunum, while the other forms appear to be absorbed by passive diffusion. K2 (made by bacterial synthesis) is actually absorbed locally in the colon, but the degree to which this occurs may be highly variable. As a fat-soluble vitamin, all three compounds of vitamin K are best absorbed in the presence of fat and bile salts. In individuals with fat malabsorption, vitamin K uptake from food may be diminished by half or more.[1] Vitamin K is delivered to the organs via circulation in very low density lipoprotein (VLDL) and low density lipoprotein (LDL). Only very small amounts of the vitamin are stored, with primary storage sites being the kidney, bone marrow, adrenal gland, and lymph nodes. Vitamin K also degrades quite rapidly. Limited storage plus rapid degradation makes the risk for deficiency in the absence of dietary intake quite high.

The primary function of vitamin K is in blood clotting. There are seven vitamin K-dependent clotting factors in the clotting cascade: factors II (prothrombin), VII, IX, and X, and proteins C, S, and Z. Interestingly, the numbered "factors" promote clotting while the lettered proteins actually inhibit clotting, resulting in a balance between the two.

Vitamin K-dependent proteins are also important to bone health. Both osteocalcin and matrix Gla protein (MGP) are vitamin K-dependent. Protein S may also play a role in bone metabolism. All three are made by osteoblasts. Studies going back more than two decades have demonstrated that vitamin K deficiency or use of vitamin K-antagonists[2] (coumadin, warfarin) can cause loss of bone mass, bone deformity (in newborns if the mother took blood thinners),[3] and increased fracture risk.[4] In soft tissues, such as arteries, protein S and MGP appear to prevent calcification, thus providing a link to cardiovascular disease as well.

Finally, there is a vitamin K-dependent protein called Gas6 that was discovered in the early 1990s. It is found in the nervous system, connective tissue, and several internal organs, and researchers believe it may play a role in both tissue development and aging.[5]

## DEFICIENCY

The best recognized problems associated with vitamin K deficiency in adults are disorders of clotting. These can range from mild to quite severe, depending on the degree of deficiency. Physical manifestations include unexplained bruising (especially excessive bruising in response to very minor trauma), bleeding gums, heavy or prolonged menses in women, nosebleeds, blood present in urine, and difficultly clotting, which may be noticed by patients in minor wounds (shaving, paper cuts) or by prolonged oozing after a blood draw or injection. Coughing or straining may produce petechiae. There may be bloody or tarry stools if there is bleeding into the digestive tract. In chronic, persistent vitamin K deficiency, bone loss and vascular calcification may also be signs.

The incidence of vitamin K deficiency is not documented after gastric bypass and is thought to be quite high after procedures like biliopancreatic diversion (BPD) and duodenal switch (DS).[6] Slater, et al., reported an incidence of 68 percent of patients experiencing vitamin K deficiency following weight loss surgery (WLS) after four years. Other causes of vitamin K deficiency in adults include liver disease (due to the inability to produce vitamin K-dependent proteins), biliary disease (as bile salts are required for absorption); use of coumarin-derived anticoagulants; use of drugs that bond bile acids or cause fat malabsorption (olestra, orlistat); and use of some antibiotics (due to loss of intestinal synthesis or possibly due to disruptions in vitamin K metabolism). Japanese research has indicated that poor diets or fasting after surgery can be a cause of vitamin K deficiency postoperatively.[7] Pregnant women who are vitamin K deficient are at risk of giving birth to babies with hemorrhagic disease and bony defects.

## LABORATORY EVALUATION

The screening tests plasma prothrombin (PT) and partial thromboplastin time both elevate with vitamin K deficiency. These tests will, however, miss subclinical deficiency.[8] Des-Gamma-Carboxy Prothrombin (also called DCP or PIVKA II—Protein Induced in Vitamin K Absence) is considered by many to be the most sensitive test, but may not be easy to obtain, and clinicians may find that the lab results take a long time (although it is good to note that Labcorp added the test in February, 2006). Plasma phylloquinone is probably the most accessible test with well established reference ranges that provide good sensitivity. The normal range is usually cited as 0.10 to 2.20ng/mL. Samples are typically frozen and foil-wrapped to protect them from degradation. Unfortunately, up to 15 percent of the population has very low to undetectable levels in blood, but normal tissue stores and function. Therefore, the best determination of vitamin K status is likely to be through measurement of PIVKA-II or by looking at phylloquinone together with PT and partial thromboplastin time (PTT).

Other tests that may hold greater potential for the future include urinary gamma-carboxyglutamic acid and undercarboxylated osteocalcin (ucOC). The latter can also be measured in serum and is thought to be a sensitive measure of tissue levels. However, if vitamin D is also deficient, ucOC may not be very useful, as vitamin D is required for osteocalcin synthesis.[9] While vitamin K deficiency is associated with changes in bone density, findings from a bone density screening would be impossible to differentiate from other factors. Fibrinogen level, thrombin time, and platelet count are typically normal in vitamin K deficiency, which helps to separate it from other clotting disorders.

## TREATMENT

Phylloquinone is the most common form of vitamin K used as a replacement. It can also be called phytonadione. Therapy can be initiated with a single intramuscular or subcutaneous injection of 10mg. Change in PT screening may be visible in 3 to 6 hours. If the deficiency is mild or subclinical, oral dosing is safest. A dose of 5 to 20mg will produce a change in PT screening in 6 to 12 hours. If there is no response, liver disease should be considered. In an incomplete response, a second dose can be given (8 to 12 hours after injection, 14 to 48 hours after oral dosing). Following this, maintenance should be implemented.

## PREVENTION AND MAINTENANCE

The daily adequate intake (AI) level for vitamin K is 90mcg for women and 120mcg for men. It is not known if this level is adequate after WLS. In other types of malabsorption (as in cystic fibrosis), daily dosing has been shown to be more effective than weekly.[10] In these cases, daily dosing of 180mcg has been shown to be effective in prevention. However, as noted above, a high rate of deficiency has been seen in procedures like DS, even at doses of 300mcg/day.[11]

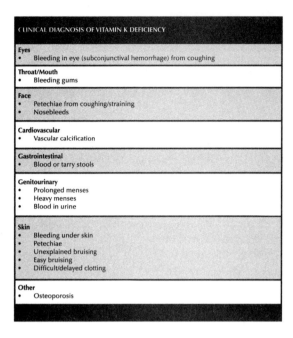

| CLINICAL DIAGNOSIS OF VITAMIN K DEFICIENCY |
| --- |
| **Eyes** |
| • Bleeding in eye (subconjunctival hemorrhage) from coughing |
| **Throat/Mouth** |
| • Bleeding gums |
| **Face** |
| • Petechiae from coughing/straining |
| • Nosebleeds |
| **Cardiovascular** |
| • Vascular calcification |
| **Gastrointestinal** |
| • Blood or tarry stools |
| **Genitourinary** |
| • Prolonged menses |
| • Heavy menses |
| • Blood in urine |
| **Skin** |
| • Bleeding under skin |
| • Petechiae |
| • Unexplained bruising |
| • Easy bruising |
| • Difficult/delayed clotting |
| **Other** |
| • Osteoporosis |

Popular products used by WLS patients contain this range, but clearly may not be adequate. The Institute of Medicine has not set a tolerable upper intake level (UL) for vitamin K. K1 and K2 are not associated with allergic reaction or toxicity even at very high doses. K3 (menadione) has been shown to produce liver damage, as it depletes glutathione.[12] Because there is only limited data, this information can only serve as a general guide, and clinicians should use lab studies and clinical evaluation to determine efficacy. It is important that oral supplements be of water dispersible forms.

Vitamin K is found in high amounts in green vegetables, carrots, parsley, egg yolk, vegetable oils, nuts, and seeds. Patients should be counseled on what foods to eat to get adequate dietary vitamin K. Freezing of foods and prolonged exposure to light diminishes vitamin K content, and low-fat foods naturally have less vitamin K than their full-fat counterparts.

It is not known whether supplementing probiotics or eating probiotic-rich foods (like yogurt or kefir) would allow for greater intestinal production of vitamin K. Dysbiosis is common after gastrointestinal surgery and has been implicated in other problems (see Chapter 2). It is also known that some classes of antibiotics (most notably cyclosporines and tetracyclines) decrease vitamin K activity and increase bleeding. Thus, it might be possible to consider probiotics as an adjunct therapy. Many preparations of live or viable cultures are available. It is best to look for strains known to establish themselves well in the digestive system (*Lactobacillus casei, L. rhamnosis, L. GG, L. acidophilus,* and Bifidus). If choosing yogurt, the cultures should be listed as well.

## INTERACTIONS AND REACTIONS

Numerous drugs interact with vitamin K. These include but are not limited to warfarin, heparin, some antibiotics, doxorubicin, some anticonvulsants (phenytoin), orlistat, olestra, cholestyramine, and laxatives. X-ray exposure and radiation deplete vitamin K levels. High-dose vitamin E may interfere with vitamin K activity. At doses of 1000IU, vitamin E has been shown to increase PIVKA-II.[13] It did not, however, alter any other vitamin-K related tests after 12 weeks. It is believed that a breakdown product of vitamin E (tocopherol-quinone) may somehow interfere with the production of some vitamin K-dependent proteins in the liver if it is present in large enough quantities. High dose vitamin A is also thought to interfere with vitamin K absorption.

## COENZYME Q10—THE "OTHER" QUINONE

Vitamin K compounds are all part of a group of organic molecules called quinines. The common link among quinones is that they contain a benzene ring with two ketone side chains. They are widespread in plants and animals with roles in photosynthesis, cellular respiration, and as both oxidants and antioxidants.

In human nutrition, we talk also about the vitamin K quinones because they are essential nutrients. However, another quinone, Coenzyme Q10 (CoQ10, ubiquinone, ubidecaquinone) has garnered much attention for its potential roles in health and disease. CoQ10 is not essential because humans can make it, but there is evidence that levels in humans are declining and this may correlate to some disease states.

CoQ10 is highly lipophilic and is found in virtually all cell and mitochondrial membranes. It is often referred to as a "metabolic antioxidant." This designation describes both its indispensable role in the creation of adenosine triphosphate (ATP) as well as in fighting lipid peroxidation (especially in low density lipoprotein [LDL] cholesterol and cell membranes).

CoQ10 is synthesized by humans in a reaction that requires both vitamin B6 and the enzyme HMG-CoA reductase. Thus deficiency of B6 could result in low levels. More importantly, there is some concern that widespread use of HMG-CoA reductase inhibitors (also known as statins) can lower CoQ10 synthesis.[1] This could create potential problems both with mitochondrial ATP synthesis and with increased production of lipid peroxides. CoQ10 depletion is significantly implicated in statin-induced myotoxicity. Studies have shown that serum levels of CoQ10 fall in stain users, and low levels on muscle biopsy are demonstrated in those who develop muscle pain with statin use.[2]

Dietary intake is thought to contribute to approximately 25 percent of human CoQ10 levels, with the main sources being animal proteins, dairy products, vegetable oils, nuts, and seeds. The optimal intake levels for humans has never been established so it is not possible to say whether most people obtain adequate amounts from diet to augment production. Supplements of CoQ10 are widely available. Again, no optimal dose has been established—studies have used doses from 30mg to as high as 1200mg.

Research on CoQ10 had focused on five areas: Cardiovascular disease, neurodegenerative disease, anti-aging, cancer, and diabetes. CoQ10 may one day prove to be a valuable therapeutic agent, beyond its general heath-supportive role. Levels of CoQ10 can be measured in serum or plasma, although the test may not be easy to obtain, and the reference ranges are not well established. Some labs give a range of 0.4 to 1.6μg/mL, while others suggest a higher range of 2.5 to 3.5μg /mL may be more beneficial.

Because of its close structural relationship to vitamin K, it is generally suggested that individuals on blood thinners not take CoQ10 without physician supervision. Despite claims, there really is not much evidence that any one form is better absorbed than another, although most sources agree that taking supplements together with some dietary fat may be beneficial.

1.    Nawarskas JJ. HMG-CoA reductase inhibitors and coenzyme Q10. *Cardiol Rev* 2005;13(2):76–9.
2.    Lamperti C, Naini AB, Lucchini V, et al. Muscle coenzyme Q10 level in statin-related myopathy. *Arch Neurol* 2005;62(11):1709–12.

## CONCLUSION

Vitamin K deficiency is most likely to be seen with significantly malabsorptive procedures, although there does appear to be a general risk after gastrointestinal (GI) surgery. Frankly, we do not know the real risk after most procedures due to lack of reporting. Bruising and bleeding gums are common complaints of WLS patients. I have often heard this dismissed by physicians as insignificant. Given the importance of vitamin K not only to clotting, but also to bone and cardiovascular disease, these complaints should likely be given more weight, and vitamin K evaluations should be performed if such clinical signs are present.

## REFERENCES

1.    Groff JL, Gropper SS, Hunt SM. *Advanced Nutrition and Human Metabolism, Second Edition.* Minneapolis, MN: West Publishing, 1995:313–19.
2.    Booth SL, Mayer J. Warfarin use and fracture risk. *Nutr Rev* 2000;58(1):20–2.
3.    Vermeer K, Jie KS, Knapen MH. Role of Vitamin K in bone metabolism. *Ann Rev Nutr* 1995;15:1–22.
4.    Caraballo PJ, Heit JA, Atkinson EJ, et al. Long-term use of oral anticoagulants and the risk of fracture. *Arch Intern Med* 1999;159(15):1750–6.
5.    Tsaioun KI. Vitamin K-dependent proteins in the developing and aging nervous system. *Nutr Rev* 1999;57(8):231–40.
6.    Slater GH, Ren CJ, Siegel N, et al. Serum fat-soluble vitamin deficiency and abnormal calcium metabolism after malabsorptive bariatric surgery. *J Gastrointest Surg* 2004;8:48–55.
7.    Usui Y, Tanimura H, Nishimura N, et al. Vitamin K concentrations in the plasma and liver of surgical patients. *Am J Clin Nutr* 1990;51(5):846–52.
8.    Suttie JW. Vitamin K and human nutrition. *J Am Diet Assoc* 1992;92(5):585–90.
9.    Takahashi M, Naitou K, Ohishi T, et al. Effect of vitamin K and/or D on undercarboxylated and intact osteocalcin in osteoporotic patients with vertebral or hip fractures. *Clin Endocrinol* (Oxf) 2001;54:219–24.
10.   Wilson DC, Rashid M, Durie PR, et al. Treatment of vitamin K deficiency in cystic fibrosis: Effectiveness of a daily fat-soluble vitamin combination. *Pediatrics* 2001;138:851–5.
11.   Slater GH, Ren CJ, Siegel N, et al. Serum fat-soluble vitamin deficiency and abnormal calcium metabolism after malabsorptive bariatric surgery. *J Gastrointest Surg* 2004;8:48–55.
12.   Nishikawa Y, Carr BI, Wang M, et al. Growth inhibition of hepatoma cells induced by vitamin K and its analogs. *J Biol Chem* 1995;270:28304–10.
13.   Booth SL, Golly I, Sacheck JM, et al. Effect of vitamin E supplementation on vitamin K status in adults with normal coagulation status. *Am J Clin Nutr* 2004;80(1):143–8.

# CHAPTER 9

# Vitamin E

Vitamin E is a fat-soluble nutrient that is actually eight compounds—four tocopherols and four tocotrienols. The synthetic dl-alpha-tocopherol (all-rac-alpha tocopherol) is also referred to as vitamin E and is found in dietary supplements and fortified foods. We will discuss the differences in these forms in greater detail toward the end of this chapter. Tocopherols are considered to be the most active of the vitamin E compounds and are found throughout the food chain in both plant and animal sources.

The primary function of vitamin E in the body is as an antioxidant. Because it is fat-soluble, it is important for preventing oxidation of fats in places like cell

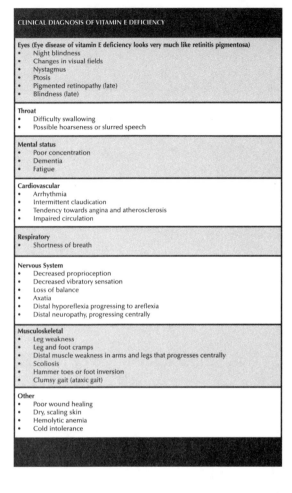

**CLINICAL DIAGNOSIS OF VITAMIN E DEFICIENCY**

**Eyes (Eye disease of vitamin E deficiency looks very much like retinitis pigmentosa)**
- Night blindness
- Changes in visual fields
- Nystagmus
- Ptosis
- Pigmented retinopathy (late)
- Blindness (late)

**Throat**
- Difficulty swallowing
- Possible hoarseness or slurred speech

**Mental status**
- Poor concentration
- Dementia
- Fatigue

**Cardiovascular**
- Arrhythmia
- Intermittent claudication
- Tendency towards angina and atherosclerosis
- Impaired circulation

**Respiratory**
- Shortness of breath

**Nervous System**
- Decreased proprioception
- Decreased vibratory sensation
- Loss of balance
- Axatia
- Distal hyporeflexia progressing to areflexia
- Distal neuropathy, progressing centrally

**Musculoskeletal**
- Leg weakness
- Leg and foot cramps
- Distal muscle weakness in arms and legs that progresses centrally
- Scoliosis
- Hammer toes or foot inversion
- Clumsy gait (ataxic gait)

**Other**
- Poor wound healing
- Dry, scaling skin
- Hemolytic anemia
- Cold intolerance

membranes and mitochondria, as well as preventing the oxidation of low density lipoproteins (LDL) circulating in the blood. Vitamin E also plays a small role in cell signaling, affecting the expression of some immune cells. It also has a role in circulation being somewhat vasodilatory, inducing nitric oxide and having some antithrombic function.

In its antioxidant role, vitamin E is called a "chain-breaking" antioxidant due to its ability to block the destructive free-radical cascade in the phospholipids membrane of human cells. Once it has done its job, however, such as donating an electron to neutralize something like a dangerous peroxyl radical, vitamin E becomes a free radical itself (the tocopherol radical). It then must contact another antioxidant (such as vitamin C or coenzyme Q10) in order to be recycled back to a harmless form. Accordingly, vitamin C must also be recycled by glutathione or lipoic acid, which must in turn be restored by nicotinamide adenine dinucleotide (NADH) or nicotinamide adenine dinucleotide phosphate (NADPH). This is important to understand since it shows that while vitamin E is a very important antioxidant, it is really at the top of a cascade. In studies examining therapeutic doses of vitamin E, it has been suggested that the rest of the cascade cannot bear the burden of tocopherol radical generated (and so on down the line). Thus, it is important that while we recognize the importance of vitamin E as an independent nutrient, we must see its overall larger place as well.

Only plants, not animals, make vitamin E. Oily plants are richest in vitamin E and provide the most bioavailable sources. Animal fats also concentrate vitamin E, and it is present in animal sources only to the degree it was present in the diet of the animal. Most vitamin E is absorbed in micellar form by passive diffusion in the jejunum. This process is dependent on bile and pancreatic enzymes, which are involved in the formation of the micelles. As there are cases of vitamin E deficiency reported in the clear absence of fat malabsorption, it is also suspected that another unidentified factor plays a role in uptake. Percent absorption of vitamin E is variable and generally decreases as dose increases. Like most fatty nutrients, vitamin E is transported in lymph. In the case of vitamin E, LDL is the carrier molecule. LDL is also responsible for the transport of vitamin E into target cells via the LDL receptor.

## DEFICIENCY

Vitamin E deficiency is generally considered to be quite rare. Findings are primarily neuromuscular and resemble spinocerebellar ataxia. Early findings may include memory changes, distal muscular weakness, loss of proprioception and balance, decreased vibratory sensation, night blindness, changes in visual fields, and diminished deep-tendon reflexes. As disease progresses, there can be frank dementia, nystagmus, blindness, retinal disease (pigmented retinopathy), ptosis, areflexia, progressive neuropathy and myelopathy, arrhythmia, and dysphagia. While early stages are reversible, late stages are not. Many clinical texts note that the symptoms can be identical to any ataxia, while eye disease can mimic retinitis pigmentosa, thus these conditions should be part of the differential diagnosis.

Vitamin E levels are not commonly evaluated after weight loss surgery (WLS), so good statistics are not available. Deficiency would be more likely to occur following procedures such as duodenal switch (DS) and biliopancreatic diversion (BPD), which produce greater malabsorption of fats. A review of 170 BPd patients (with and without DS) found a deficiency rate of four percent after four years.[1] Thus we must conclude that the risk is small and patients must, in general, be absorbing vitamin E well compared to other fat soluble nutrients, such as vitamin A, where the same review found a 52-percent rate of deficiency after 12 months).

Known risk factors for vitamin E deficiency are short-bowel syndrome, abetalipoproteinemia, cystic fibrosis, cholestatic liver disease, and malabsorption. As vitamin E is so widespread in the diet, the greatest risk with WLS appears to be the degree of malabsorption.

## LABORATORY EVALUATION

Vitamin E is easily measured in serum or plasma.[2] Serum levels below 11.6μmol/L (5μg/mL) are considered too low.[3] Since LDL cholesterol is the major carrier of vitamin E in the body and travels primarily in plasma, an alternate method of evaluation is to look at the ratio of plasma tocopherol to cholesterol. Ratios lower than 2.2 are equated with deficiency.

Other possible measurements of vitamin E status include erythrocyte hemolysis, breath testing for gasses, and measurements in lymphocytes, erythrocytes, or platelets. Erythrocyte hemolysis is a simple test for vitamin E that is predicated on the fact that the membranes of red blood cells become fragile when vitamin E levels are low. This correlates very well with serum vitamin E levels. Hemolysis can be induced in dilute hydrogen peroxide. The limitation is that one must use extremely fresh blood cells. When vitamin E levels are low, there is greater reduction of lipid peroxides in the body. Byproducts of lipid peroxidation include the gasses pentane and ethane, which can be evaluated in breath. While both gasses do correlate with low vitamin E levels, the tests are not readily available, samples can be challenging to collect, and low levels of other antioxidants can also increase lipid peroxidation. Malondialdehyde levels also rise with impaired antioxidant status, including vitamin E. Elevations have been shown to correspond to deficiency in children, but not in adults. Some data exists to indicate that vitamin E levels in erythrocytes and especially platelets may provide an earlier and more sensitive measure of vitamin E status. These procedures are somewhat tricky to perform and are not yet in common use.

Vitamin E in specimens is highly sensitive to light and heat-induced oxidation. Care should be taken to protect samples. It is recommended that samples be frozen or shipped on ice. Some labs recommend handling under low light and/or wrapping the tube in foil.

Electrodiagnosis can be useful in the diagnosis of vitamin E-induced neuropathy. Electromyogram (EMG) findings should be unremarkable, which is different from other nutritional neuropathies. Changes in somatosensory evoked response (SEP) and somatosensory evoked potentials (SSEP) are present with the former being reduced and the latter reflecting a delay in central conduction.

## TREATMENT

Some references list vitamin E in milligrams, other in international units (IU). To dose vitamin E products, it is important to understand the difference. Most vitamin E that is supplemented is alpha-tocopherol. The synthetic and natural forms are used interchangeably, but are not equivalent in their activity level. Natural vitamin E, which will be listed on a product label as d-alpha-tocopherol or tocopheryl (or as RRR-alpha-tocopherol) has a much higher vitamin E activity than the synthetic form (seen on a label as dl-alpha-tocopherol or all-rac-alpha-tocopherol). Margaret Traber, PhD, the esteemed vitamin E researcher, gives the equivalents as follows:[4]

RRR-alpha-tocopherol (natural or d-alpha-tocopherol):
- IU x 0.67 = mg RRR-alpha-tocopherol.
- Example: 100IU = 67mg

all-rac-alpha-tocopherol (synthetic or dl-alpha-tocopherol):
- IU x 0.45 = mg RRR-alpha-tocopherol.
- Example: 100IU = 45mg

Large ranges are often cited for replacement of vitamin E in deficiency states. The *Merck Manual* cites a range of 15 to 25mg/kg/day for malabsorption syndromes. For a 150-pound person, this would be a range of 680IU to about 1150IU of natural vitamin E. Some references cite a larger range of 200IU to 3600IU.[5] Doses for neuropathy start at 100mg/kg/day (this is 6800IU for a 150-pound adult). This should be given in divided doses, with doses tapering when symptoms begin to subside. Alternately, injections of vitamin E can be given. The water-miscible forms are preferred in malabsorption as they have demonstrated better uptake. Many sources state that recovery from neuropathy is often incomplete despite recovery of laboratory values.

## PREVENTION AND MAINTENANCE

The recommended daily allowance (RDA) for vitamin E is 15mg (22.5IU) of natural vitamin E. Prevention of deficiency and maintenance of normal status will be dependent on the procedure performed. It is not known whether there is any need to supplement above the RDA in Roux-en-y (RNY) patients. With DS, an exact quantity is also not known to prevent

**FOOD FOR THOUGHT**

Just as the B vitamins work synergistically in the body, so too are antioxidants interdependent. Vitamin E, CoEnzyme Q10, and vitamin C are closely related to each other in their physiological functions. Some studies have indicated that supraphysiologic doses of vitamin E can do harm. This may be, in part, due to the generation of levels of tocopherol radical sufficient to overwhelm the system. While unsupported by clinical data, it may be wise to consider that if supplementing high-dose vitamin E, the antioxidants that support the recycling of the tocopherol radical should be supplemented as well.

deficiency. The study cited above found a four-percent occurrence of deficiency and used a dose of 60IU of vitamin E. In practice, many programs utilize products with much higher levels in the range of 150 to 600IU, sometimes in addition to levels in a multivitamin.

In general, these levels would be considered safe. One thousand milligrams (1500IU) is considered by the Institute of Medicine to be the tolerable upper limit (UL) for vitamin E. This is based on the level least likely to cause red cell hemolysis and bleeding. Levels over 1600IU/day may inhibit vitamin K-dependant clotting. Similar levels have also been shown to increase oxidation of LDL cholesterol.[6] Daily use of levels greater than 2000IU (higher than the UL) is associated with an increased risk of death.[7] It is difficult, however, to know how this data would apply in cases of surgical malabsorption. Of final note, some studies in both humans and animals have demonstrated impaired thyroid function at doses of 600IU/day. Because many patients with obesity have concurrent thyroid dysfunction, this may be worth taking into account when considering dosage.[8] Lastly, there is some evidence that the disease retinitis pigmentosa may be accelerated by high-dose vitamin E therapy.

Vitamin E is well distributed throughout the human diet. The best sources include oils, such as olive, soybean, and safflower; nuts and seeds; and avocado. Sweet potatoes, mangos, and asparagus are also high in vitamin E, but virtually all fruits, vegetables, grains, and seeds have some vitamin E. Some studies have suggested that vitamin E in foods is able to produce much higher blood levels than the nutrient alone.[9] It may thus make sense to counsel at-risk patients to look for vitamin E-fortified foods in addition to supplemental sources.

## INTERACTIONS AND REACTIONS

Vitamin E does have drug interactions. Because of the potential for increased bleeding, concurrent use of blood thinners or aspirin therapy should be closely monitored. The higher the vitamin E level, the greater the risk. For this reason, patients on vitamin E therapy are also generally asked to discontinue taking products containing vitamin E at levels higher than the RDA two or more weeks prior to a surgical procedure. There is some evidence that vitamin E inhibits the uptake in the brain of tricyclic antidepressants, antipsychotics in the phenothiazine class, and propranolol. The fat-blocking drugs orlistat and olestra can decrease absorption of vitamin E. Since orlistat has been approved for over-the-counter use, patients who take it should be monitored for vitamin E deficiency.

## CONCLUSION

Vitamin E is an important antioxidant that plays a vital role in human health. While deficiency seems to be rare, there is a risk with significant malabsorptive procedures. In terms of testing, regular evaluations of vitamin E levels likely make sense only in those patients who are at greatest risk. Alternately, patients who present with symptoms of neuropathy that is not due to other causes should be evaluated for vitamin E status.

## REFERENCES

1.  Slater GH, Ren CJ, Siegel N, et al. Serum fat-soluble vitamin deficiency and abnormal calcium metabolism after malabsorptive bariatric surgery. *J Gastrointest Surg* 2004;8:48–55.
2.  Horwitt MK, Harvey CC, Dahm CH Jr, Searcy MT. Relationship between tocopherol and serum lipids for determination of nutritional adequacy. *Ann N Y Acad Sci* 1972;203:223–6.
3.  Higdon J. Vitamin E. Available at: http://lpi.oregonstate.edu/infocenter/vitamins/vitaminE/index.html. Access date: November 2004.
4.  Kaplan GE. Vitamin E Deficiency. Available at: http://www.emedicine.com/MED/topic2383.htm. Access date: March 2004.
5.  Reaven PD, Wiztum JL. Comparison of supplementation of RRR-alpha-tocopherol and racemic alpha-tocopherol in humans. Effects of lipid levels and lipoprotein susceptibility to oxidation. *Arterioscler Thromb* 1993;13:601–8.
6.  Miller ER, Pastor-Barriuso R, Dalal D. Meta-analysis: High-dosage vitamin E supplementation may increase all-cause mortality. *Ann Intern Med* 2005;142(1):37–46.
7.  Tsai AC, Kelley JJ, Peng B, Cook N. Study on the effect of megavitamin E supplementation in man. *Am J Clin Nutr* 1978;31:831–7.
8.  Leonard SW, Good CK, Gugger ET, Traber MG. Vitamin E bioavailability from fortified breakfast cereal is greater than that from encapsulated supplements. *Am J Clin Nutr* 2004 Jan;79(1):86–92.

# CHAPTER 10

# Calcium

alcium is the most abundant mineral in the human body. It plays a vital role in body structure, but has other critical functions in human physiology. Ninety-nine percent of whole body calcium is incorporated into the structure of bones and teeth. The remaining one percent is distributed throughout the body. Many cells contain calcium channels in their membranes. Calcium ions moving through these channels trigger nerve impulses, muscle contraction (including in the heart), blood vessel contraction and relaxation, and secretion of endocrine hormones. Calcium is also part of the clotting cascade, interacting with vitamin K in the activation of clotting factors.

Calcium from foods and some types of dietary supplements must become ionized in an acid medium in order to be absorbed in the small intestine. It is believed that the calcium must be in an acid medium for approximately one hour for this to occur. Some forms of calcium bound to highly soluble ligands can be absorbed in non-ionized forms.

Calcium is absorbed by more than one mechanism throughout the small intestine. Active transport occurs in the duodenum and proximal jejunum. Transport in the duodenum is thought to be most efficient. Passive diffusion of calcium can occur anywhere in the small intestine, but the ileum is the most abundant area. Dietary factors can have a great influence over calcium bioavailability. Dietary oxalate can significantly bind to calcium, making it unavailable for absorption. Oxalate is found in many vegetables, such as spinach, sweet potatoes, and beans, as well as berries and chocolate. Phytate, mostly found in grains, can impair absorption to a much lesser degree. Magnesium and calcium will compete for absorption if both are present in substantial amounts. Phosphorus at a level greater than calcium may impair calcium balance. However, this is a complex relationship and it will be covered in more depth under Interactions. Large amounts of sodium and protein both increase calcium loss. Caffeine can significantly increase calcium loss in the urine and gut. Steatorrhea will cause decreased calcium absorption when undigested fats bind with calcium in the gut, creating soaps that cannot be absorbed. Typically, with steatorrhea, vitamin D is also poorly absorbed, leveling a double blow to bone health. This can be a significant problem with weight loss surgery (WLS) patients and will be discussed later.

Active transport is dependant on both dietary intake and the needs of the body at the time of intake. This process is highly vitamin D-dependent.[1] Passive diffusion takes place between the cells of the intestinal lumen (rather than through them). It is completely dependent on the amount of ionized calcium present in the gut and is not dependent on vitamin D status. Some passive diffusion can also occur in the colon, and under the right circumstances this can account for up to four percent of calcium absorption.[2] There is some indication that individuals with less absorption of calcium in the proximal intestine will be able to absorb more calcium from the colon.

About half of absorbed calcium travels unbound in the body. Of the other half, most is bound to albumen or other proteins, and a smaller fraction is complexed to a ligand like citrate or phosphate.

It is important to know that calcium within the body is tightly regulated. Parathormone, calcitonin, and vitamin D are the primary regulatory agents, but sex hormones, adrenal hormones, and factors like IGF-1 and leptin have influence over bone mineralization or loss as well. Because of the vital functions that calcium regulates, any changes in blood calcium levels above or below the desired range signal the calcium regulatory system to remove calcium from bone, absorb more or less calcium from the gut, and excrete more or less calcium in the urine. Thus, when dietary calcium levels are low or absorption is poor (or both), the body will simply remove calcium from bone to keep blood levels in the desired range. In many cases, this is perfectly painless and causes few dramatic symptoms until bone loss is severe.

## DEFICIENCY

In discussing calcium deficiency, we need to touch on both hypocalcemia and metabolic bone disease. Isolated hypocalcemia tends to occur with disorders of calcium metabolism, the most common of which is hypoparathyroidism. This condition will not be discussed here since it is not believed that this occurs as a result of weight loss surgery (WLS). Other causes of hypocalcemia that can occur with WLS include low intake, low protein, malabsorption, hypo or achlorhydria, hypomagnesemia, and vitamin D deficiency. Metabolic bone disease includes the conditions of osteoporosis, osteomalacia, and hyperparathyroidism. All three of these conditions are known to occur after WLS.

Mild or even moderate hypocalcemia can be completely asymptomatic. Neuromuscular irritability can manifest with spontaneous muscle cramping, paraesthesia in the fingers (and sometimes toes), numbness of the fingers and hands, and loss of sensation around the mouth. Patients may report that muscles are stiff, painful, and cramp easily with minimal work. They may also have unexplained gastrointestinal cramps. Difficult breathing can result from bronchospasm, and patients with asthma may report more frequent, hard to control attacks. Hypotension can result in faintness, increased spontaneous sweating can occur, and there can be difficulty swallowing. If a patient has a history of epilepsy, there may be an increased frequency of seizure activity.

The two classic diagnostic signs of hypocalcemia are Chvostek's sign and Trousseau's sign. Chvostek's sign is evoked by tapping firmly on the face just anterior to the ear (approximately 2cm) and below the zygomatic process (approximately 0.5cm). This corresponds to a superficial location of cranial nerve VII (the facial nerve). An alternate site is one-third the distance down an imaginary line drawn from the most prominent point of the cheekbone to the ipsilateral corner of the mouth. A positive Chvostek's sign involves contraction of the muscles innervated by cranial nerve VII—especially those around the mouth and eye. One may also observe twitching of the nose and spasm of the other facial muscles. Trousseau's sign can also be elicited in a physical exam. To perform the test, a blood pressure cuff is placed in the normal position for measuring blood pressure. The cuff is then inflated to just above systolic pressure in order to occlude the brachial artery. In hypocalcemia, this will cause the following within two to three minutes: Flexion of the wrist, flexion of the thumb against the palm, and hyperextension of the fingers. Trousseau's sign is considered to be the most sensitive clinical feature of hypocalcemic tetany. However, it can also be seen with hypomagnesemia, so one cannot make a diagnosis based solely on positive physical exam.

Bone is the storage pool for almost all calcium in the body, and bone loss will result from chronic deficiency. Bone loss secondary to chronically low calcium can result in skeletal problems including fracture. Fractures are often associated with a major trauma, such as falls, but the incident may also be minor and unmemorable. Vertebral compression fractures may present with acute, localized spinal pain and spasm of the paraspinal muscles. Fractures of the hip can cause localized pain, decreased range of motion, and radiating pain similar to sciatica. If bone loss has been ongoing for many years, loss of height, thoracic kyphosis ("dowager's hump), and lumbar flattening may be observed. Fractures can also occur at other sites of injury—the wrist, shoulder, and ribs are common locations. Other chronic manifestations of low calcium include dry skin, brittle hair and nails, poor dental health, psoriatic skin lesions, itching, anxiety, agitation, depression, hypertension, and increased risk for colon cancer.

All forms of surgery have been shown to produce increased bone turnover and loss of bone mass,[3] some of which is inevitable with massive weight loss. Still, from a review of current published literature, it is hard to establish the true incidence by procedure. This is further confounded by other unknown influences on data, including bone health prior to surgery, peak bone mass achieved, lifetime diet and exercise habits, sex hormone levels, and

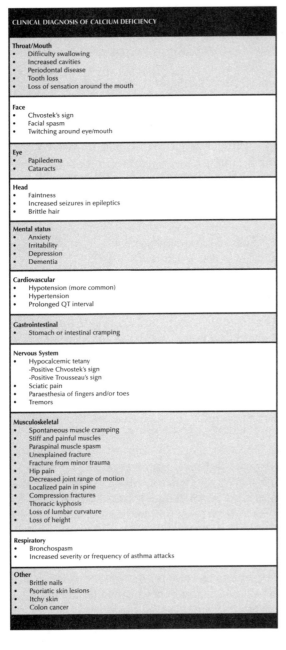

| CLINICAL DIAGNOSIS OF CALCIUM DEFICIENCY |
| --- |
| **Throat/Mouth**<br>• Difficulty swallowing<br>• Increased cavities<br>• Periodontal disease<br>• Tooth loss<br>• Loss of sensation around the mouth |
| **Face**<br>• Chvostek's sign<br>• Facial spasm<br>• Twitching around eye/mouth |
| **Eye**<br>• Papiledema<br>• Cataracts |
| **Head**<br>• Faintness<br>• Increased seizures in epileptics<br>• Brittle hair |
| **Mental status**<br>• Anxiety<br>• Irritability<br>• Depression<br>• Dementia |
| **Cardiovascular**<br>• Hypotension (more common)<br>• Hypertension<br>• Prolonged QT interval |
| **Gastrointestinal**<br>• Stomach or intestinal cramping |
| **Nervous System**<br>• Hypocalcemic tetany<br>  -Positive Chvostek's sign<br>  -Positive Trousseau's sign<br>• Sciatic pain<br>• Paraesthesia of fingers and/or toes<br>• Tremors |
| **Musculoskeletal**<br>• Spontaneous muscle cramping<br>• Stiff and painful muscles<br>• Paraspinal muscle spasm<br>• Unexplained fracture<br>• Fracture from minor trauma<br>• Hip pain<br>• Decreased joint range of motion<br>• Localized pain in spine<br>• Compression fractures<br>• Thoracic kyphosis<br>• Loss of lumbar curvature<br>• Loss of height |
| **Respiratory**<br>• Bronchospasm<br>• Increased severity or frequency of asthma attacks |
| **Other**<br>• Brittle nails<br>• Psoriatic skin lesions<br>• Itchy skin<br>• Colon cancer |

medication use. One study found that 66 percent of women had evidence of bone loss 3 to 5 years after Roux-en-y (RNY) surgery.[4] Hypocalcemia, hypovitaminosis D, and hyperparathyroidism have been reported in 48 percent, 63 percent, and 69 percent of patients with WLS four years post-operatively, respectively.[5] A one-year study in adjustable gastric band (AGB) patients following numerous markers (including vitamin D, parathyroid hormone [PTH], telopeptides, and dual energy x-ray absorptiometry [DEXA]) found that there was significant evidence of negative bone remodeling in the absence of secondary hyperparathyroidism. Researchers found considerable bone loss primarily at the hip with increased telopeptide levels (indicating active loss of bone).[6] As there is no malabsorption in AGB, it must be assumed that accelerated bone loss here is restricted to decreased dietary intake and weight loss itself.

## LAB EVALUATION

There is no simple assessment for calcium balance in the body, and several methods must be employed simultaneously to get a good picture of what is happening in the body. Clinicians must also consider the weight loss surgical procedure performed, nutritional supplementation, diet, age, gender, medication use, and activity levels, which can help guide the selection of laboratory assessments.

Because the body will demineralize bone to maintain normal serum calcium levels, serum measurement does little to assess nutriture. These levels are, however, commonly used to diagnose hypocalcemia. A serum below 8.2mg/dL or a serum ionized calcium below 4.4mg/dL confirms hypocalcemia, but does not indicate the cause. In WLS patients, the most common causes that can be found with laboratory diagnosis are vitamin D deficiency followed by magnesium and protein deficiencies. If hypocalcemia is suspected from history and physical exam, it is probably wise to evaluate for magnesium and D at the same time. It is clinically valuable to evaluate intact PTH (iPTH), which is elevated with low vitamin D and may also be altered with magnesium deficiency. It is also common practice to rule out renal failure and pancreatitis, which can be done by assessing creatinine, creatine kinase, and amylase levels.

Since low protein can be a cause of hypocalcemia and occurs with some forms of WLS (especially biliopancreatic diversion [BPD]and duodenal switch [DS]), albumen levels can be assessed in these patients. If found to be low, a corrected calcium (also called calcium corrected for albumen) should be calculated.[7] This estimates what serum calcium levels would be if there were adequate albumen. Finally, serum phosphate levels can be useful. If low, this can be associated with vitamin D deficiency or low intake; they can be elevated with renal failure and primary hypoparathyroidism.

As the skeletal system is such a rich storage bank for calcium, the body can be depleting calcium without ever developing hypocalcemia. Osteoporosis is a thinning of bone tissue resulting in increased fracture risk; osteomalacia is a softening of bone due to abnormal/reduced bone mineralization, usually caused by vitamin D deficiency. Both are common after WLS. Because these conditions are often silent, producing few if any clinical symptoms until they are quite advanced, it is important to assess bone health in WLS patients. The most accepted test for the evaluation of bone density is DEXA, a low-energy X-ray technique that evaluates bone in the hip and lumbar spine. Results of a DEXA are reported as a T-score (rating of patient's bone density against that of a young adult). T-scores below 2.5 are diagnostic for osteoporosis; T-scores between 1 and 2.5 indicate osteopenia. DEXA findings may also be abnormal with osteomalacia. Often in this case, there is selective or greater bone loss at the hip as compared to the spine. Newer assessments of bone density include the p-DEXA (p for peripheral), which examines the bones of the forearm, and heel ultrasound. These are often less costly, which may make them more accessible to some patients. Data on these tests is not as well substantiated as with DEXA. Computed tomography (CT), magnetic resonance imaging (MRI), and single-photon emission computed tomography (SPECT) techniques also exist for the evaluation of bone density.

Bone is active tissue that is created and destroyed throughout life. Laboratory studies can also assess markers of bone turnover. This can be helpful both in initial assessment and in tracking response to treatment or intervention. The most commonly used measurements are collagen cross links, which include pyridinolines and C- and N-telopeptides. These can be assessed in serum or urine. Elevated levels are found in bone loss before findings are detectable on DEXA. Hydroxyproline can also be measured in urine, and levels are elevated with bone loss. These markers are very useful in establishing treatment response as they can change rapidly. Markers of bone formation are also available in a limited capacity. These include bone-specific alk phos and type-1 procollagen.

Electrocardiogram and electrocardiograph studies can also be ordered in hypocalcemic patients to evaluate for arrhythmias. A prolonged QT time may also be observed. Further, clinicians should not forget causes of bone loss unrelated to WLS. Depending on the age, sex, and health of the patient, it is important to consider sex hormones, thyroid hormones, medications, and general risk factors for bone loss that exist outside of those created by surgery.

## TREATMENT

Treatment of acute or severe hypocalcemia may require intravenous (IV) repletion in an inpatient setting. Acute hypocalcium usually involves a serum calcium below 7mg/dL. This is usually done with 100 to 200mg of elemental calcium from calcium gluconate. This should be given slowly over about 20 minutes with close attention to cardiac reactivity. Following this initial dose, or in less severe cases, a calcium infusion can be initiated at 0.5mg/kg/hour (up to 2mg/kg/hour is sometimes used) until the patient can be stabilized. Co-existing problems like low magnesium are usually addressed at the same time. Patients are usually kept under close watch until they can be stabilized with an oral preparation.

Chronic or mild hypocalcemia should be treated with oral calcium. Vitamin D is usually required as well, and magnesium may also be indicated if low. Other underlying causes, such as low protein, must be addressed. The doses used for treatment are usually in the range of 1500 to 2000mg of elemental calcium per day in divided doses. With RNY and DS, there may be concern of bioavailability of some forms like calcium carbonate. Calcium carbonate normally combines with hydrochloric acid in the stomach to form calcium chloride, which is ultimately well absorbed. This is unlikely to occur after RNY. A small comparative study between the two forms was conducted in postoperative RNY patients and also concluded that calcium citrate was significantly more bioavailable in this population.[8] For this reason, calcium citrate is preferred for both treatment and prevention. Different calcium salts contain different levels of elemental calcium. Supplements should be labeled showing the amount of elemental calcium followed by the source or sources, i.e., 1000mg calcium (citrate), 500mg calcium (carbonate), or 1200mg calcium (citrate, lactate, carbonate). Sometimes only the quantity of the total complex is listed. Common forms of calcium contain the following percentages of elemental calcium:

- Carbonate: 40 percent
- Citrate: 21 percent
- Lactate: 13 percent
- Gluconate: 9 percent

Preparations from shell, dolomite, or bone meal should be avoided due to possible problematic lead and aluminum levels.

Many drugs are now available for the treatment of osteoporosis. These include antiresorptive medications, hormone therapies, PTH, and calcitonin. These should only be administered after the cause of bone loss has been determined such that an appropriate therapy can be selected. If vitamin D deficiency is present, it should be corrected prior to administration of a bisphosphonate so as not to exacerbate or induce hypocalcemia.[9]

## PREVENTION AND MAINTENANCE

Prevention is the best tool to guard against hypocalcemia and metabolic bone disease. Patients should be counseled about diet, exercise, smoking, and other lifestyle factors that affect calcium status and bone health. Dietary supplements of calcium are a very common recommendation after WLS. The recommended daily allowance (RDA) for calcium is 1000mg for adults up to age 50, and then rises to 1200mg. The common recommendation for post-menopausal women is 1500mg.

After AGB, adequate amounts of calcium to account for dietary restriction should be given. This can be estimated by having the patient keep a detailed three-day diet log. The form of calcium (i.e., citrate, carbonate, lactate, etc.) is less important to AGB patients as they have no malabsorption. Calcium is commonly recommended as a postoperative supplement in the range of 1000 to 1500 milligrams per day. Higher doses up to 2000 milligrams are sometime advised after DS. Calcium is best taken in divided doses of no more than 500mg at a time, and should be taken separately from iron supplements to avoid interference with iron absorption.

A challenge with calcium supplementation tends to be the number of pills that need to be taken daily. Patients should be encouraged to establish a routine with supplementation. For some patients, chewable or liquid preparations may be more advantageous. Understanding the serious nature of deficiency and bone loss sometimes helps with adherence. Both patients and clinicians should understand that bone loss occurs for many reasons and that it may develop despite best efforts at risk reduction. The goal, therefore, is to manage risk by combined efforts through diet, lifestyle modifications, use of supplements, and regular laboratory assessments to catch problems that may arise at the earliest possible time.

Diet is an important source of calcium. Dairy products, tofu, and fortified drinks (juice, soy milk, rice milk) are by far the best sources. Patients troubled by lactose intolerance can be instructed in the use of lactase, which usually allows for normal consumption of dairy foods. Beans and dark green vegetables also have substantial calcium, but it is much less bioavailable due to phytates and oxalates as discussed above. Fish in which the bones are edible (sardines, anchovies, canned salmon) are outstanding sources of calcium with high bioavailability.

## EXCESS AND TOXICITY

There is very little toxicity caused by oral calcium. The Institute of Medicine set the tolerable upper limit (UL) at 2500mg. The most common problems associated with this level are gastrointestinal in nature and include constipation, nausea, vomiting, dry mouth, and loss of appetite. There is also increased risk of kidney stone formation in patients who are stone formers. Patients who have histories of kidney stones should be instructed to take calcium with food rather than between meals.

## INTERACTIONS

Calcium has many known interactions with both nutrients and drugs. Food interactions have already been covered. Iron absorption can be significantly impaired by large doses of calcium or by calcium-rich foods. Co-consumption of iron with a high calcium load can decrease iron absorption by up to 62 percent.[10] Phosphorus can both cause increased calcium excretion in the gut and reduce calcium loss in the urine. A chronic high-phosphorus, low calcium diet can result in elevated PTH and overall net bone loss. Yet phosphorus is an abundant mineral in bone and is incredibly important for bone health. A balanced ratio of calcium to phosphorus (close to 1:1) has been suggested as best for bone health. The richest sources of phosphorus in the American diet are meats, high protein foods, and grains. Meats usually have a calcium to phosphorus ratio of 1:10 to 1:20. A single soda may have 20 to 50mg of phosphorus and no calcium. Dairy products, such as a cup of milk, are almost a perfect balance. Excessive intakes of sodium and caffeine also increase calcium loss from the body. Magnesium is required for PTH secretion. If it is low, as it often is in cases of low calcium, then PTH may not rise as high as expected and will not function correctly in the body. Zinc and calcium also have reported interactions. High calcium levels taken concurrently with zinc can decrease zinc absorption by as much as 50 percent,[11] yet in individuals with low dietary intake of calcium, zinc supplementation has been shown to decrease calcium uptake.[12] Ultimately, when using supplemental calcium for long-term risk reduction, it is important to ensure that other minerals are adequately represented. Separately, elevated homocysteine (which can occur with low B12 or folate) is also associated with increased risk of osteoporosis and fracture for reasons that are not yet well understood.[12]

Some medications are not adequately absorbed in the presence of calcium. These include many antibiotics (tetracycline, doxycycline, minocycline, and quinolones) and thyroid hormones. Some cardiac medications (such as propranolol and its derivatives and calcium channel blockers) may be less effective in those taking calcium supplements. There are also many drugs that contribute to calcium loss. Individuals who need to be on calcium supplements and are also taking prescription medication should consult with their pharmacists.

## CONCLUSION

Calcium deficiency can pose both an acute risk and a long-term health threat. Assessment of calcium nutriture can be a challenge for clinicians and may take a multidisciplinary effort, especially in difficult cases. Acute deficiency of calcium is not nearly as common as metabolic bone disease, which is a systemic problem going far beyond simple nutrition. Risk reduction through use of supplements and regular lab evaluations are an important part of helping patients retain bone integrity as they age. Clinicians must keep in mind that calcium does not make up the whole picture when it comes to bone health, and it is important to consider the range of possibilities when approaching treatment of calcium deficiency. This cycle is explained in greater detail in Chapter 7.

## REFERENCES

1. Pansu D, Bronner F. Nutritional aspects of calcium absorption. *J Nutr* 1999;129:9–12.
2. Coates PS, Fernstrom JD, Fernstrom MH, et al. Gastric bypass surgery for morbid obesity leads to an increase in bone turnover and a decrease in bone mass. *J Clin Endocrinol Metab* 2004;89(3):1061–5.
3. Goode LR, Brolin RE, Chowdhury HA, Shapses SA. Bone and gastric bypass surgery: Effects of dietary calcium and vitamin D. *Obes Res* 2004;12(1):40–7.
4. Slater GH, Ren CJ, Siegel N, et al. Serum fat-soluble vitamin deficiency and abnormal calcium metabolism after malabsorptive bariatric surgery. *J Gastrointest Surg* 2004;8:48–55.
5. Pugnale N, Giusti V, Suter M, et al. Bone metabolism and risk of secondary hyperparathyroidism 12 months after gastric banding in obese pre-menopausal women. *Int J Obes Relat Metab Disord* 2003;27(1):110–6.
6. Corrected calcium (mg/dL) = measured total Ca (mg/dL) + 0.8 (4.0 - serum albumin [g/dL]), where 4.0 represents the average albumin level.
7. Chang CG, Simms T, Adams-Huet B, et al. A comparison of the absorption of calcium citrate and calcium carbonate after Roux-en-Y gastric bypass. Clinical Proceedings of the 21st Annual Meeting of the American Society of Bariatric Surgeons. Available at: http://www.asbs.org/html/pdf/asbs_abstract_booklet.pdf. Access date: January 19, 2005.
8. Rosen CJ, Brown S. Severe hypocalcemia after intravenous bisphosphonate therapy in occult vitamin D deficiency. *N Engl J Med* 2003;348(15):1503–4.
9. Cook JD, Dassenko SA, Whitaker P. Calcium supplementation: Affect on iron absorption. *Am J Clin Nutr* 1991;54:266S–73S.
10. Wood RJ, Zheng JJ. High dietary calcium intakes reduce zinc absorption and balance in humans. *Am J Clin Nutr* 1997;65(6):1803–9.
11. Spencer H. Minerals and mineral interactions in human beings. *J Am Diet Assoc* 1986;86(7):864–7.
12. van Meurs JB, Dhonukshe-Rutten RA, Pluijm SM, et al. Homocysteine levels and the risk of osteoporotic fracture. *N Engl J Med* 2004;350(20):2033–41.

# CHAPTER 11

# Magnesium

Magnesium is the fourth most abundant mineral in the human body. It is the second most abundant extracellular ion and has vast physiologic roles in health. Magnesium is involved in over 300 metabolic reactions affecting almost every organ of the body. Approximately 60 percent of body magnesium plays a structural role as part of bone. The remaining 40 percent is found in muscle, other soft tissues, and intracellular fluids.

Magnesium is essential to the binding of adenosine triphosphate (ATP) to phosphate groups, making it vital to cellular energy production. It is involved in the Krebs cycle; beta-oxidation; creatine formation;

| CLINICAL DIAGNOSIS OF MAGNESIUM DEFICIENCY (ALSO SEE CALCIUM DEFICIENCY AND THIAMINE DEFICIENCY) |
|---|

**Eyes**
- Blurred vision
- Nystagmus

**Throat/Mouth**
- Difficultly swallowing
- Espohageal spasm

**Face**
- Chvostek's sign
- Facial spasm
- Twitching around eye/mouth

**Head**
- Focal Seizure
- Grand Mal Seizure
- Dizziness
- Vertigo
- Migraine

**Mental status**
- Depression
- Lethargy
- Irritability
- Personality changes
- Delirium
- Coma (severe)

**Cardiovascular**
- Dysrhythmia
- Ventricular tachycardia
- Torsades de pointes
- Atrial fibrillation
- Atrial flutter
- Angina
- Ischemic heart disease
- Hypertension
- Atherosclerosis
- Vasospasm
- Prolonged QT and PR intervals
- Wide QRS complex
- ST depression

**Gastrointestinal**
- Constipation
- Gastrointestinal spasm
- GI colic

**Respiratory**
- Shortness of breath
- Bronchospasm

**Nervous System**
- Tremor
- Ataxic gait
- Positive Chvostek's sign (see calcium)
- Positive Trousseau's sign (see calcium)
- Signs and symptoms of hypocalcemic tetany (see calcium)
- Can coexist with thiamine deficiency and have overlapping symptoms
- Paresthesias (mostly fingers, can be toes)

**Musculoskeletal**
- Muscle weakness
- Muscle spasm and cramping
- Fasiculations
- Myopathy
- Fibromyalgia
- Restless Leg Syndrome
- Osteoporosis

**Metabolic**
- Hypocalcemia
- Hypokalemia
- Hyponatremia
- Hypophosphatemia
- Acidosis
- Hyperglycemia

**Other**
- PMS
- Menstrual cramping
- Preeclampsia of pregnancy

deoxyribonucleic acid (DNA) and ribonucleic acid (RNA) synthesis and transcription; cardiac muscle contraction; synthesis of some proteins, fats, and carbohydrates; and the formation of cyclin adenosine monophosphate (cAMP) and glutathione. In addition to bone, magnesium also plays a structural role in cell membranes. It is important both to cell signaling and cell migration. Moreover, it regulates the transport of calcium and potassium as well as some other ions across cell membranes—giving magnesium a vital role in the control of nerve impulse and muscle contraction.

Despite its crucial roles in the human body, we do not fully understand the digestion and absorption of magnesium. The importance of an acidic milieu to magnesium solubility and release from its bound state from food is not fully understood. While this is believed to be of importance as with calcium and iron, no studies have been conducted in humans. Comparative studies of magnesium oxide versus citrate, for example, show the latter to be significantly more bioavailable in humans,[1] which is thought to be due to the latter being soluble across a wide pH range. Magnesium oxide, on the other hand, only achieves slightly better than 40 percent solubility even at optimal stomach acidity.

Absorption of magnesium occurs throughout the small intestine and is concentrated in the distal jejunum and the ileum. Some absorption can also occur in the colon. Vitamin D has a positive influence on magnesium absorption, and fat malabsorption causes the formation of soaps in the gut, preventing absorption. Absorption ultimately occurs by both active and passive transport. More than half of circulating magnesium is unbound. The remainder is either bound to protein or a ligand, such as citrate. Approximately 65 percent of total body magnesium is stored in bone. Roughly an additional 35 percent is found in muscle. The rest is distributed in cell membranes, biological molecules, proteins, and in the extracellular matrix.

## DEFICIENCY

Normally, magnesium deficiency is an extremely rare condition. But in select conditions, such as malabsorption postoperatively, protein deficiency, chronic diarrhea, eating disorders, alcohol abuse, or diabetes, it can occur. Despite discussion among clinicians, studies or case reports of magnesium deficiency are virtually absent in published weight loss surgery (WLS) literature. Twenty years ago, Halverson, et al., reported a deficiency rate of 34 percent in Roux-en-y (RNY) patients more than one year postoperative.[2] The exceptions are reports in the now obsolete jejunoileal bypass (JIB),

| MAGNESIUM SALTS AND THEIR % ELEMENTAL MAGNESIUM | |
|---|---|
| **MAGNESIUM SALT** | **PERCENT MAGNESIUM** |
| Oxide | 60% |
| Hydroxide | 42% |
| Citrate | 16% |
| Lactate | 12% |
| Sulfate | 10% |
| Glycinate | 10% |
| L-aspartate | 9.9% |
| Gluconate | 5.9% |

If the magnesium products you are using do not list the amount of elemental magnesium in the preparation, you may need to calculate it.

12.2mg of elemental magnesium is equal to 1mEq.

where magnesium deficiency was commonly reported. Magnesium deficiency after RNY is less likely than after biliopancreatic diversion (BPD) or duodenal switch (DS) due to the length of bowel bypassed relative to the sites of optimal uptake. Moreover, steatorrhea, vitamin D loss, and protein loss all increase the likelihood of magnesium deficiency. Postoperatively, dehydration is a significant contributing factor in magnesium deficiency. Dehydration can cause an increase in aldosterone, which in turn causes magnesium to be excreted in much larger quantities by the kidneys. Less magnesium means less parathyroid hormone (PTH), which means less active vitamin D. As vitamin D is then needed for both calcium and magnesium absorption, this can set up a vicious cycle. Patients on medications that increase magnesium excretion (such as thiazide, loop diuretics, and aminoglycosides) are at even greater risk. For reasons not completely understood, African Americans appear to have a significantly higher risk for developing magnesium deficiency when compared to other populations,[3] so clinicians may have a higher index of suspicion in these patients.

There is not a singular clinical picture of low magnesium. This is both because it plays such diverse roles in the body and because it rarely occurs in isolation. In acute deficiency, the clinical picture reported often is indistinguishable from calcium deficiency. Symptoms of thiamine deficiency can also overlap. This is because magnesium is required for transforming thiamine into the biologically active thiamine pyrophosphate (TPP). There can be muscle weakness, pain, spasm, tremor, cramping, nausea, loss of appetite, difficulty swallowing, paresthesias, fasciculations, dizziness, blurred vision, depression, irritability, lethargy, insomnia, and personality changes. As with calcium deficiency, Trousseau's and Chvostek's signs may be positive. Tachycardia, hypertension, and arrhythmias may be observed. Mild to moderate and chronic deficiencies are often asymptomatic. The most common systems affected are the cardiovascular and nervous systems. Metabolic changes can also be seen. But in these cases, there may only be findings of chronic disease, such as hypertension, high cholesterol, diabetes, migraine, arrhythmia, ischemic heart disease, asthma, fibromyalgia, pre-menstrual syndrome, restless leg syndrome, and osteoporosis. Patients may report poor exercise tolerance or shortness of breath with minimal exertion. Preeclampsia of pregnancy is also correlated with magnesium deficiency, and magnesium is increasingly used in the therapeutic treatment of this condition.

## LAB EVALUATION

Serum magnesium is the most common value used to assess status. It is limited, however. If a low serum magnesium level is present, then there is good assurance that intracellular levels are low and the patient is truly deficient. Unfortunately, serum levels can also be normal in the case of intracellular depletion.[4] This is because magnesium in serum represents only around one percent of total body magnesium, and there are many biological controls regulating this value. Red blood cell (RBC) magnesium screening has become much more readily available and is thought to be an accurate reflection of intracellular levels. This test is considerably more expensive than serum magnesium, however. Clinicians suspecting magnesium deficiency but finding normal serum levels or those treating patients with hypocalcemia or thiamine deficiency may consider RBC magnesium important for accurate diagnosis and treatment.

## TREATMENT

Correction of underlying problems, such as dehydration, should be considered in addressing hypomagnesemia. Because intravenous (IV) administration of magnesium is dangerous, it is usually reserved for acute symptomatic cases and is given in an inpatient setting. The IV form used is magnesium sulfate, and the total dose is usually given slowly over several days. Mild to moderate deficiency (serum levels in the range of 1.2 to 1.7mg/dL), especially in cases where serum magnesium is normal, should be approached with oral supplementation. A typical dose would be 50 to 100mg of elemental magnesium given three times daily. Doses of less than 350mg/day are generally well tolerated. There are many magnesium salts available, including oxide, carbonate, hydroxide, citrate, chloride, gluconate, and chloride. As with calcium, some forms like citrate and gluconate are considerably more soluble. Chloride and lactate also appear to be good choices.[5] This makes them a better choice for patients with WLS. These forms also tend to be easier on the digestive system, producing less diarrhea. Magnesium-based antacids are not well absorbed and should not be used for treatment. Patients may tolerate higher doses if they are given at night on an empty stomach. This is advantageous because transit time is slower, allowing for greater absorption. If patients have steatorrhea, magnesium should be taken on an empty stomach or with a low fat/fat-free meal.

## PREVENTION AND MAINTENANCE

The recommended daily allowance (RDA) for magnesium is 420mg/day for men and 320mg/day for women. In the standard American diet, typical intakes fall about 25 percent below this.[6] Whole grains, nuts, seeds, beans, avocados, corn, oysters, and green vegetables are good dietary sources. Patients following high protein, low carbohydrate eating plans that are common after WLS may get less magnesium than the average person based on their food selections.[7] For this reason it is likely that supplemental magnesium at least to the level of the RDA would be of benefit. Many patients who undergo WLS have a history of diseases that are associated with magnesium deficiency. Nearly 40 percent of people with diabetes have been found to have low magnesium,[8] and rates are also high in heart disease, hypertension, and asthma. It is not known whether weight loss would help to correct this or if it is part of an underlying predisposition to all of these conditions. Still, it may be that some patients need higher levels of magnesium to help balance their personal biochemistry. There is no tolerable upper limit (UL) for magnesium from food sources. From supplements given in addition to diet, the UL is set at 350mg/day for adults. Multivitamins often contain very little magnesium, so this should be taken into consideration when selecting products. Sometimes magnesium is found in calcium supplements. A level of 100 to 250mg of supplemental magnesium (over and above dietary intake) is probably very reasonable for prevention so long as it does not cause a laxative effect.

## EXCESS AND TOXICITY

As magnesium is a laxative, the most common side effect of too much is diarrhea. In true hypermagnesemia, there can be lethargy, reduced consciousness, abnormal heart rate and rhythm, kidney dysfunction, severe hypotension, sleepiness, weakness, and, if severe, death. The upper level of 350mg is for supplements in addition to diet, and is the highest amount known to pose virtually no risk of side effects in adults.

## INTERACTIONS

We have already discussed the interactions between magnesium, calcium, vitamin D, and thiamine. Magnesium also influences the homeostasis of potassium in the body, and deficiencies of the two often coexist in patients taking diuretics. Vitamin B6 increases magnesium uptake into the cells.

Some potassium-sparing diuretics also spare magnesium, so it is usually advisable to avoid supplements of either in patients using these drugs. Magnesium can reduce the absorption of tetracyclines, cimetidine, chloroquine, misoprostol, nitrofurantoin, quinolones, and several other drugs. In patients taking regular prescriptions or needing antibiotic therapy, it is best to inquire about potential drug interactions if magnesium is also required.

## CONCLUSION

Despite few reports in literature, there is likely more magnesium deficiency after WLS than we know. Part of the problem is that diagnostic screening tests can miss mild to moderate cases, and deficiency can mimic other problems and go unrecognized. Magnesium should be considered in cases as discussed above with calcium deficiency and thiamine deficiency. Patients with fat malabsorption, taking diuretics, of African American descent, or with chronic diseases associated with low magnesium should have a higher index of suspicion should symptoms arise. Annual screening for magnesium is probably a good idea for patients with BPD/DS, but is hard to advise in those with other procedures. In RNY, a test can be done reflexively if an associated deficiency is found or if there are suggestive symptoms. Overall, more data is needed to understand the long-term potential for WLS patients to develop low magnesium.

## REFERENCES

1.  Lindberg JS, Zobitz MM, Poindexter JR, et al. Magnesium bioavailability from magnesium citrate and magnesium oxide. *J Am Coll Nutr* 1990;9:48–55.
2.  Halverson JD. Micronutrient deficiencies after gastric bypass for morbid obesity. *Am Surg* 1986;52(11):594–8.
3.  Jing MA, Folsom AR, Melnick SL. Associations of serum and dietary magnesium with cardiovascular disease, hypertension, diabetes, insulin and carotid arterial wall thickness: The ARIC study. *J Clin Epidemiol* 1995;48:927–40.
4.  McLean RM. Magnesium and its therapeutic uses: A review. *Am J Med* 1994;96:63–76.
5.  Firoz M, Graber M. Bioavailability of US commercial magnesium preparations. *Magnes Res* 2001;14:257–62.
6.  Food and Nutrition Board. Institute of Medicine. Magnesium. *Dietary Reference Intakes: Calcium, Phosphorus, Magnesium, Vitamin D, and Fluoride.* Washington, DC: National Academy Pres, 1997:190–249.
7.  Bowman SA. An evaluation of high protein diets: Their energy content and nutrient profile. Presented at the Society of Nutritional Education 35th Annual Meeting. St. Paul, MN: July 27-31, 2004. Vol. 35, No. 1.
8.  Tosiello L. Hypomagnesemia and diabetes mellitus. A review of clinical implications. *Arch Intern Med* 1996;156(11):1143–8.

# CHAPTER 12

# Iron

ron is an essential trace mineral that functions in literally hundreds of proteins and enzymes in the human body. To fairly discuss all of its functions would take a small book. When most clinicians think about iron they think about anemia. This is primarily because of the role iron plays in hemoglobin, the compound in red blood cells that carries oxygen to all the cells in the human body. A similar iron-containing compound called myoglobin stores oxygen in muscle cells. Other iron-dependent chemicals help the body sense when oxygen levels are too low.[1] Iron-containing enzymes around the body and especially in the immune system act both as oxidizing agents (to kill bacteria) and as antioxidants. Deoxyribonucleic acid (DNA) synthesis also depends on an iron-containing enzyme, making iron vitally important to growth, development, and tissue repair. Finally, there are the iron-containing cytochromes. These compounds are important to metabolism and detoxification of both endogenous and exogenous chemicals, alcohol, drugs, toxins, and pollutants. Other important cytochromes are involved in the synthesis of adenosine triphosphate (ATP).

Like most trace minerals, iron has both nutritional and non-nutritional states. For iron, the nutrient forms are the ferrous (3+) and ferric (3+) states. Dietary iron occurs in two forms—heme and non-heme. Heme iron occurs only in animals. Non-heme occurs in both plants and animals. The forms are treated differently in digestion and absorption. Heme iron is by far easier for humans to absorb as it is not bound in the same manner as non-heme iron. Most of the heme iron we eat is in myoglobin and must be hydrolyzed by hydrochloric acid (HCl) and pepsin in the stomach. Once this occurs, heme can be absorbed intact in the small intestine.

Non-heme iron absorption is more work. Again, hydrolysis must occur, but freed non-heme iron must be exposed to acid to maintain it in a ferrous form. This is a challenge in the small intestine where the pH is generally alkaline. In alkaline pH, there is a high risk of non-heme iron forming insoluble compounds and becoming impossible to absorb. Natural substances, such as vitamin C, organic acids (citric, lactic, tartaric), some sugars, and sugar alcohols, can significantly enhance non-heme iron absorption. Additionally, concurrent ingestion of non-heme iron together with meat significantly improves uptake. Use of a combination of iron with an enhancing agent can improve absorption by four times or more over baseline.[2] This can be very useful in both prevention and treatment of iron deficiency.

Likewise, iron is sensitive to other factors in the diet, which can seriously impair absorption. Concurrent calcium consumption can decrease iron absorption from 49 percent[3] to 62 percent[3] (at doses of 600mg). Same goes for calcium-rich foods. Polyphenols in coffee, black tea, berries, and some vegetables can bind strongly to iron and inhibit absorption.[4] Evidence indicates that vitamin C counteracts this reaction. Phytic acid found in many beans and grains can also strongly inhibit iron absorption. This likely accounts for the reduced iron absorption seen with concurrent ingestion of soy foods. Zinc and copper are additionally thought to compete with iron for uptake in the small intestine.

Iron is preferentially absorbed in the proximal duodenum. The upper jejunum can also absorb iron relatively well. To a much lesser degree, the rest of the small intestine and the colon can absorb some iron.

Absorption of iron is also dependant on iron stores. If stores are adequate, typically no more than 1mg per day will be absorbed. When stores fall, this can rise as high as 6mg per day. Heme iron is directly absorbed by passive diffusion. Non-heme iron is taken up by a divalent metal transporter by active transport. Once taken up by the cell of the gastrointestinal tract, ferroprotein, apoferritin, and apotransferrin carry it through the mucosal cells. The incorporation of iron into these carrier molecules forms ferritin and transferrin, respectively. Some iron may remain here and be used locally or stay in storage as ferritin.

While critical to human life, iron is a potent oxidizing agent, and the body does not want to have free iron in circulation. Virtually all iron in the body is carried bound to a protein or in hemoglobin. Transferrin is the primary carrier and is found in plasma. All cells that require iron have specialized receptors for transferrin-iron complexes such that they can absorb circulating iron. Iron taken into cells is then held by ferritin. Most iron in the body is meticulously

## HEREDITARY HEMOCHROMATOSIS (HH)

Hereditary hemochromatosis (HH) is a common genetic abnormality resulting in over-accumulation of iron in the body. In the US, it is estimated that around 3 in every 1000 adults has HH, although it is much higher for those of European descent (perhaps 1 in every 200). Ten percent of the adult population is thought to carry the genetic mutation. Unless people know the condition runs in their family and they have undergone early genetic screening, onset of symptoms is typically insidious over many decades. Most people are diagnosed in their 40s or 50s, even if they have had symptoms for many years. The delay is because of how HH presents. This condition has no distinct characteristics of its own, but rather symptoms develop based on where iron accumulate. The most common early complaints of HH are arthritis and fatigue. HH can look like almost any type of arthritis, but is often mistaken for gout. Hyperpigmentation of sun-exposed skin or skin folds occurs in almost 90 percent of patients; hair loss, including body hair, occurs in over 60 percent of patients. Patients may also have thick, dry, scaly patches of skin (ichthyosis). Heart disease (especially palpitations and arrhythmia), impotence, liver disease, hypothyroidism, and diabetes are also symptoms of HH. Since many of these conditions are also seen with obesity, HH may be completely overlooked as a possible cause. Three case reports on HH in postoperative weight loss surgery (WLS) patients were presented in *Obesity Surgery* in 2004. All patients actually did well—developing neither iron deficiency nor overload. Clinicians should be suspicious of HH in patients who present with consistently high ferritins and/or transferrin saturation. Typically, ferritin is over 200 in premenopausal women and over 300 in post-menopausal women and men. Transferrin saturation is often elevated as well. Transaminases and blood sugar are also commonly elevated (although it is not known if the latter might normalize after WLS).

recycled, but some is lost. Daily average iron loss is about 1mg through sweat, urine, and skin shedding. Menstruating women lose the most—about 16 additional milligrams per month on average, but the loss can be as high as 100mg in women with heavy or prolonged menses.

## DEFICIENCY

Iron deficiency is a decrease in iron stores, usually defined by low ferritin. Iron deficiency anemia is a progression of iron deficiency whereby red blood synthesis is impaired due to lack of available heme. The body stores between 2 and 4 grams of iron. If stores are high, and loss is small, it may take years for a deficiency to show up, even with malabsorption. On the other hand, if stores are low and there is malabsorption, low intake, or loss (e.g., due to menstruation), deficiency can develop rapidly. This is because more than 95 percent of daily iron needs come from iron recycling, and only a very small amount is contributed by dietary intake.

Iron deficiency usually develops slowly. In the absence of anemia, there may be no complaints or only vague complaints like fatigue. Leg cramping, restless legs, easy muscle fatigability, ice eating (pagophagia), and pica are also seen in subclinical deficiency. Ferritins below 40ng/mL are associated with hair loss.[5]

| CLINICAL DIAGNOSIS OF IRON DEFICIENCY |
| --- |
| **Eyes** |
| • Conjunctival pallor |
| • Bluish sclera |
| **Throat/Mouth** |
| • Sore/swollen tongue |
| • Angular cheilitis |
| • Difficulty swallowing |
| • Loss of appetite |
| **Face** |
| • Pallor |
| **Head** |
| • Hair loss/telogen effluvium |
| • Headache |
| • Lightheadedness |
| • Fainting with anemia |
| **Mental status** |
| • Fatigue—often the first and most prominent symptom |
| • Irritability—also common |
| • Depression |
| • Loss of appetite |
| • Difficult concentration |
| • Slowed cognitive function |
| • "Brain Fog" |
| **Cardiovascular** |
| • Tachycardia |
| • Rapid pulse |
| **Gastrointestinal** |
| • Splenomegaly |
| • Loss of appetite |
| **Musculoskeletal** |
| • Overall physical fatigue |
| • Weakness with minimal work |
| • Restless Leg Syndrome |
| • Leg cramping |
| **Hematologic** |
| • Normocytic anemia progressing to Microcytic, hypochromic anemia |
| • Decreased MCV, MCH, MCHC |
| • Low ferritin and transferrin saturation |
| • High TIBC |
| **Other** |
| • Ice eating |
| • Pica |
| • Nail spooning or vertically ridged nails |
| • Persistent coldness |
| • Sensitivity to cold |

As deficiency progresses to anemia, fatigue will progress. Irritability is a common complaint. Physical fatigue in response to minimal work is often reported, as is shortness of breath. There can be pallor of the skin and mucous membranes. An easy place to observe this in individuals of all skin types is the conjunctiva of the eye. Patients may develop difficult swallowing, loss of appetite, sore/swollen tongue, and angular cheilitis. Hair loss (telogen effluvium) and brittle nails are also associated with iron deficiency. Koilonychia, a condition where nails become thin and concave (spooning) and develop vertical ridges, may be observed. Headache and lightheadedness can be reported. Tachycardia and rapid pulse can be observed, and there can be an enlargement of the spleen. Other symptoms can include difficult concentration, slowed cognitive function,[6] persistent coldness, and decreased immune function, which may show as more frequent or prolonged illnesses. There is also an association between iron deficiency and depression.[7]

Iron deficiency has been reported with all forms of weight loss surgery (WLS). Deficiency is relatively common post Roux-en-y (RNY) and duodenal switch (DS), with incidence increasing over time. Studies cite rates of 16 to 26 percent after one year.[8] Longer-term studies have shown incidence as high as 47 percent.[9] Iron deficiency develops with RNY and DS due to reduced hydrolysis in the stomach coupled with bypass of the primary absorptive surface in the duodenum—in other words there is both malabsorption and maldigestion. Menstruating women and those who become pregnant are at greatest risk. Iron status does not generally appear to be a problem after adjustable gastric banding (AGB), as both stomach and small intestines are preserved. However, a single study of 80 patients presented at the 2004 meeting of the American Society for Bariatric Surgery (ASBS) reported anemia in 53 percent of patients and iron deficiency in 72 percent of patients 5 to 18 months after AGB placement.[10] Clearly this data indicates a need for further research into iron nutrition and AGB.

## LAB EVALUATION

Laboratory evaluation of iron status is important both for prevention and treatment. Because symptoms can be absent or vague, regular screening of iron status is recommended. As iron absorption is impaired with most procedures, it is best to catch patients when stores are falling, rather than later when anemia is present; regular screening should allow most cases to be caught early.

Iron deficiency is staged in three phases. In the first phase, only stores are depleted. In this phase, serum ferritin is the most sensitive and specific test. Serum ferritin is a simple, inexpensive screen with well established reference

| | Iron Labs in Deficiency or Overload States | | | |
|---|---|---|---|---|
| | Iron Overload | Normal | Iron Deficiency | |
| | | | Without Anemia | With Anemia |
| Marrow Iron Stores | ↑ | normal | ↓ or absent | absent |
| Serum Ferritin | ↑ | normal | ↓ | ↓ |
| Serum Iron | ↑ | normal | ↓ | ↓ |
| Transferrin Saturation | ↑ | normal | ↓ | ↓ |
| TIBC | ↓ | normal | ↑ | ↑ |
| Hb | normal | normal | normal | ↓ |
| MCV | normal | normal | normal | ↓ |

ranges. Low levels are specific to iron deficiency, thus helping to differentiate iron-deficiency anemia from other causes. Ranges may vary from lab to lab, and are usually given by gender. Typical ranges are 22 to 322ng/mL in men and 10 to 291ng/mL in women. Iron deficiency is usually defined by ferritin below 12. However, iron depletion is considered to start at 20ng/mL. As ferritin can be elevated with chronic inflammation (with conditions such as rheumatoid arthritis, lupus, hepatitis, or cancer), the cut-off for deficiency may rise as high as 70ng/mL. In these cases, it is probably best to use additional criteria for diagnosis. The combination of ferritin with total iron binding capacity (TIBC) and serum iron will confirm virtually any case of iron deficiency but may not catch these early cases if significant inflammation is present. In the first phase of deficiency, erythrocyte protoporphyrin also rises due to impaired hemoglobin synthesis. This also occurs before the development of anemia. This test is probably unnecessary if you are measuring ferritin.

In the second phase of deficiency, serum iron levels and mean corpuscular volume (MCV) begin to fall, marking the onset of anemia. TIBC also rises in this phase, as do transferrin levels because the body is trying to absorb more iron. Serum iron levels between 60 and 115ug/dL are a sign of depletion, as is TIBC between 360 and 390ug/dL. Ferritins in this phase are usually below 10. Sometimes microcytosis appears in this phase. If you are monitoring serum iron, be sure to draw levels fasting in the morning as there is up to a 30-percent diurnal variation.

Finally, in the third stage, anemia develops. This may start with a normocytic anemia, but will develop into a microcytic, hypochromic anemia. With full-blown iron deficiency anemia, MCV and mean corpuscular hemoglobin (MCH) are low; hematocrit and hemoglobin are both low; serum iron is below 40; ferritin is below 10; TIBC is above 390; and transferrin saturation is below 15. In addition, platelet counts may be elevated, and sideroblasts fall below 10 percent.

Even though WLS patients have an obvious means for the development of iron deficiency, it may still be important to rule out other causes. Thus, clinicians should ask patients about heavy menses, hemorrhoids, and history of nonsteroidal anti-inflammatory drug (NSAID) use. Tests such as fecal occult blood, upper and lower GI studies, and urinalysis may be necessary to completely rule out bleeding.

## TREATMENT

The major question with iron deficiency and WLS may well be, "When do you intervene?" If we are using ferritin as a reference range, we see that there is a gap between deficiency and depletion. As stated above, 20ng/mL is considered depletion. If we wait until patients have iron-deficiency anemia, it may take longer and be more difficult to correct the problem. At least one study in postoperative WLS patients has demonstrated that correction of iron deficiency postoperatively is not fully successful.[11]

Typical treatment for correcting iron deficiency is high-dose oral iron therapy. Commonly recommended doses are 100 to 200mg of elemental iron per day in divided doses. At least one small study of postoperative WLS patients demonstrated that a dose of 100mg of iron (50mg of elemental iron as ferrous sulfate) was successful in treating iron deficiency, but not necessarily anemia, in menstruating women.[12] In another study, investigators supplemented anemic postoperative patients with 150mg of ferrous gluconate (in three divided doses) with and without the inclusion of vitamin C and found that both groups responded to therapy, but the results were somewhat better with the inclusion of vitamin C.[13] The treatment phase of this latter study followed patients closely for two months, then recontacted them again nearly two years later. Despite the fact that anemia and iron deficiency had improved significantly in the intervention, many patients discontinued treatment on their own and subsequently became anemic. To a lesser degree, patients who reported continuation of iron therapy also developed some anemia.

Still, it appears that in many patients, a good response to oral iron therapy can be obtained. Clinicians should be aware that a typical time to see response with oral iron in iron deficiency anemia (improvement in HCT and HGB, for example) is at 1 to 2 months. Iron stores may not show significant improvement for 3 to 6 months. As an early marker to see response to therapy, a reticulocyte count can be useful. If a patient is responsive to treatment, there should be an increase in reticulocytes at 7 to 10 days. If patients are responding, even slowly, oral therapy remains the treatment of choice, due to its relative safety.

Adherence is a serious challenge with oral iron therapy. Iron commonly produces digestive side effects, such as nausea and constipation, that can be very uncomfortable. Nonadherence with therapy is a well-accepted cause of persistent anemia. Clinicians should forewarn patients about intestinal side effects of iron therapy. It many be necessary to try more than one preparation in patients who experience problems. Taking iron with a small amount of food can help to minimize side effects, and in this case, patients should be counseled about avoiding foods that impair iron absorption when taken together. This includes advising patients to take calcium two hours away from taking iron and avoiding ingestion of coffee or black tea one hour before and after a dose. Some medications also impair iron absorption (see Interactions). Regular, frequent follow-up with iron-deficient patients will help to foster adherence.

One question with oral iron therapy is, "Should you dose every day?" With the administration of therapeutic levels of iron, some significant portion can be retained by enterocytes. It has been demonstrated that this locally retained iron decreases further GI uptake. Thus some studies have indicated that supplementation every 5 to 7 days (the approximated turn-over rate for new enterocytes) provides equivalent or somewhat better results to daily dosing, with better adherence and fewer complaints of GI symptoms.[14,15] This method has not been studied in WLS patients, but may be worth consideration in some patients.

There is also evidence that concurrent supplementation with vitamin A may be more effective than supplementing iron alone. In countries where both deficiencies are common, greater improvement in iron deficiency is seen when both nutrients are supplemented versus iron alone, even in the absence of proven vitamin A deficiency.[16] This is likely due to vitamin A's role in the transport of iron into the hemoglobin of developing RBCs. It is not known whether combined supplementation would benefit WLS patients with iron deficiency. Levels used in humans have been around 10,000IU, which is generally considered safe for adults. This addition may be worth trying in more difficult cases of iron deficiency.

Some patients may not be responsive to oral iron therapy or may just be poor candidates (demonstrated nonadherence, ongoing GI challenges with high-oral dosing, severe anemia). In these cases, iron dextran given intravenously is the treatment of choice. While riskier than oral therapy, it is preferred over allowing a patient to remain iron deficient. Because of the risk of allergic reaction and anaphylaxis, a test dose is always recommended. This is usually done with a slow IV push (approximately one minute) of 0.5mg iron dextran. The patient should then be observed for an hour with monitoring of heart rate, respiration, and blood pressure as well as physical appearance. If there is no reaction, therapy can be initiated. Reactions can also be delayed, so patients need to be educated to look for fever, chills, rash, and signs of anaphylaxis. Mild symptoms can usually be managed with an NSAID or by predosing with prednisone or methylprednisone. Epinephrine, diphenhydramine, and IV hydrocortisone should be kept at hand whenever one is using IV iron therapy. IV iron dose is determined by a calculation as follows:

- Mg iron = [0.3 x wt (lbs) x 100 (14.8 – current hemoglobin)]/14.8. Note: If patient is still obese, it is recommended to use lean body mass over actual body weight. There are online calculators that do this automatically. A good one can be found at: http://www.globalrph.com/irondextran.htm.
- If the response to the test dose is favorable, it can be given as a total dose diluted in normal saline. This is typically done over 4 to 8 hours with the iron diluted in 250 to 1000mg of normal saline.

- Alternately, the total dose can be divided into 100mg increments and given as a series of small pushes or infusions every 1 to 3 days. In patients who are mildly reactive, this is probably preferred. Overall, the total infusion is preferred by most experts.[17]
- Although iron can be given intramuscularly by the Z-track method, this is painful, hard to perform, and frequently results in tattooing and allergic reactions.

Response of patients to iron replacement is the same regardless whether it is given orally or parenterally.[18] Recovery should be monitored closely. If a patient has an incomplete response to an infusion, it may be repeated after 3 to 6 months.

## PREVENTION AND MAINTENANCE

There is no agreement about iron prophylaxis in the WLS community. Some programs give iron preventively, some give none, and some only give it to premenopausal or pregnant women. As mentioned above, rates of iron deficiency are quite high, and deficiency can occur even with supplementation. However, small studies have demonstrated efficacy in preventing deficiency, especially in menstruating women. As there is no current standard of practice, this section will merely serve to help clinicians make a choice.

The recommended daily allowance (RDA) for iron is 18mg for women and 8mg for men up to the age of 50. Over the age of 50, it is 8mg for men and women. It is important to note that the reason the RDA for women drops after age 50 is because this is an approximation of menopause. If a woman has undergone a hysterectomy or premature menopause, it is likely that her iron requirements are less. The RDA in pregnancy and lactation are 27mg and 9mg, respectively.

The concern with preventive iron therapy is that iron is toxic. Despite its importance to human health, it has a very narrow therapeutic window, and conditions like colon cancer and some forms of heart disease are tied to excessive use of iron in the lack of proven need. Additionally, since iron competes with smaller trace elements in the body, like copper and zinc, unnecessary dosing with levels above the daily requirement may result in iatrogenic deficiency of another mineral (see the Chapter 14 for a discussion of this). Finally, iron tends to produce side effects, especially in the digestive system, and this may result in increased patient complaints and nonadherence with other recommendations.

Because intestinal absorption of iron is significantly impaired after malabsorptive procedures, it might be best to consider some intervention, such as closer dietary monitoring or increased supplementation, before patients fall into a state of depletion. A ferritin level of 50 is often given as a healthy goal for those with hemochromatosis; some references cite 100±60 as "ideal," making 40 the bottom of the normal range. Studies in otherwise healthy individuals find mean serum ferritins of around 94 for men and 34 for women.[19] Since a ferritin of 20 is considered depletion and normal appears to start somewhere between 34 and 50, it might be good to consider intervention in this range. Early intervention might be as simple as counseling patients on dietary iron intake, advising them to take a supplement with the RDA of iron, and closer monitoring.

As noted above, menstruating women are at greatest risk for iron deficiency, and we do have some evidence of the level of iron that can be effective in prevention. The dose used in this study was 100mg of elemental iron (as ferrous sulfate).[20] This is a relatively high dose and we do not know if a lower dose would have also proven effective. This level also did not prevent anemia, which might raise the question of whether it might have contributed to another anemia of a nutrient like copper.

Unfortunately, the reality is that we really do not have an answer to the question of how to best prevent either iron deficiency or anemia after WLS. Dietary monitoring and regular lab evaluations are always warranted. Supplementation with RDA levels of iron is considered to be safe and could be good assurance. The Institute of Medicine sets the tolerable upper limit (UL) at 45mg of elemental iron per day for all adults based primarily on intestinal toxicity. Whether or not this has bearing in WLS is not known, but it is all we have.

Good dietary sources of iron include meat, fish, shellfish, poultry, egg yolk, dried fruits, molasses, kidney beans, lentils, tofu, cashews, and dark green leafy vegetables. Keep in mind, however, that animal sources are much superior to plant sources. Supplements come in a variety of forms, such as sulfate, fumarate, gluconate, bis-glycinate, carbonyl, and citrate. They vary in how well they are tolerated, and patients may need to try more than one form. It is generally not advised that patients who have undergone RNY or DS use slow, sustained, or time-released preparations; even though they tend to decrease digestive upset, they are not designed to be broken down in a shortened digestive system. Products also come in chewable, tablet, and liquid forms. Many patients avoid liquids due to tooth staining. Some preparations are available blended with vitamin C.

## EXCESS/TOXICITY

Gastrointestinal irritation is the most common adverse effect of iron supplementation and can include nausea, vomiting, indigestion, constipation, or diarrhea. Symptoms of chronic toxicity can include fatigue, joint and muscle pain, depression, heart palpitations, and mouth pain. There may be GI bleeding. If abnormally high ferritin or other iron labs are observed, one may need to consider an iron overload disorder (see sidebar Hereditary Hemochromatosis). Acute iron overdose is one of the more common causes of accidental overdose death in children. For this reason, iron products are sold in safety-seal packaging and should be placed out of reach of children. In adults, acute toxicity usually involves ingestion of a dose of iron greater than 40mg/kg. A single dose of 200+ mg/kg can be fatal. Signs and symptoms of acute toxicity usually start with acute, often severe GI symptoms: Nausea, vomiting, severe and bloody diarrhea, abdominal pain. Fluid loss and bleeding can be severe enough to cause shock. These symptoms can be followed by metabolic and cardiac abnormalities and multiple organ failure. For this reason, acute iron overdose is a medical emergency.

## INTERACTIONS

There are many drug, nutrient, and dietary interactions with iron. Iron can decrease the absorption of tetracycline, thyroid, bisphosphonates, levadopa, methyldopa, fluoroquinolones, and penicillimine. Iron absorption can be decreased by any acid-reducing medication, calcium, digestive enzymes, cholestyramine, chloramphenicol, and some fiber supplements. Gout medications may increase iron storage and toxicity. Absorption of copper, zinc, selenium, and vitamin E may be decreased by high iron intake. For dietary interactions, please refer to the section on absorption. It is advisable that anyone taking prescription medications plus iron supplements consult his or her doctor or pharmacist for possible interactions.

## CONCLUSION

Prevention and treatment of iron deficiency is still not entirely understood in relation to WLS. When one couples issues regarding prophylaxis with the challenges of treatment, this is possibly the best argument available for insisting that patients have regular follow up and regular lab studies. More studies should be done to help establish whether prophylaxis is effective and establish the minimum effective dose for prevention. Clinicians should give careful consideration to the issue of when they begin to intervene, especially how early intervention should begin. I personally recommend not allowing ferritin levels to drop below 20. Additionally, working with deficient and anemic patients to maximize adherence should help to reduce the number of severely anemic patients.

## REFERENCES

1.  Jaakkola P, Mole DR, Tian YM, et al. Targeting of HIF-alpha to the von Hippel-Lindau ubiquitylation complex by O2-regulated prolyl hydroxylation. *Science* 2001;292(5516):468–72.
2.  Monsen ER, Balintfy JL. Calculating dietary iron bioavailability: Refinement and computerization. *J Am Diet Assoc* 1982;80(4):307–11.
3.  Cook JD, Dassenko SA, Whittaker P. Calcium supplementation: effects on iron absorption. *Am J Clin Nutr* 1991;53:106–11.
4.  Food and Nutrition Board, Institute of Medicine. Iron. *Dietary reference intakes for vitamin A, vitamin K, boron, chromium, copper, iodine, iron, manganese, molybdenum, nickel, silicon, vanadium, and zinc.* Washington DC: National Academy Press, 2001:290–393.
5.  Rushton DH. Nutritional factors and hair loss. *Clin Exp Dermatol* 2002;27(5):396–404.
6.  Groner JA, Holtzman NA, Charney E, Mellits ED. A randomized trial of oral iron on tests of short-term memory and attention span in young pregnant women. *J Adol Health* 1986;7:44–8.
7.  Masse PG, Roberge AG. Relationship between oral contraceptives, iron status, and psychoaffective behaviour. *J Nutr Med* 1991;2:273–81.
8.  Brolin RE, Leung M. Survey of vitamin and mineral supplementation after gastric bypass and biliopancreatic diversion for morbid obesity. *Obes Surg* 1999;9(2):150–4.
9.  Brolin RE, Gorman RC, Milgrim LM, et al. Multivitamin prophylaxis in prevention of post-gastric bypass vitamin and mineral deficiencies. *Int J Obesity* 1991;15:661–7.
10. Vemulapalli P, McGinty A, Lopes J, et al. Nutritional deficiencies in laparoscopic gastric banding. Clinical Proceedings of the 21st Annual Meeting of the American Society for Bariatric Surgeons. Available at: http://www.asbs.org/html/pdf/asbs_abstract_booklet.pdf. Access date: January 19, 2005.
11. Brolin RE, Gorman RC, Milgrim LM, et al. Multivitamin prophylaxis in prevention of post-gastric bypass vitamin and mineral deficiencies. *Int J Obesity* 1991;15:661–7.
12. Brolin RE, Gorman JH, Gorman RC, et al. Prophylactic iron supplementation after Roux-en-Y gastric bypass: A prospective, double-blind, randomized study. *Arch Surg* 1998;133:740–4.
13. Rhode BM, Shustik C, Christou NV, MacLean LD. Iron absorption and therapy after gastric bypass. *Obes Surg* 1999;9(1):17–21.
14. Ridwan E, Schultink W, Dillon D, Gross R. Effects of weekly iron supplementation on pregnant Indonesian women are similar to those of daily supplementation. *Am J Clin Nutr* 1996;63:884–90.
15. Thu BD, Schultink JW, Dillon D, et al. Effect of daily and weekly micronutrient supplementation on micronutrient deficiencies and growth in young Vietnamese children. *Am J Clin Nutr* 1999;69:80–6.
16. Miller J. Vitamin A, iron, and anemia: From observation to hypotheses. *Nutrition Bytes* 1998;4(2)Article 5. Available at: http://repositories.cdlib.org/uclabiolchem/nutritionbytes/vol4/iss2/art5.
17. Auerbach M, Witt D, Toler W, et al. Clinical use of the total dose intravenous infusion of iron dextran. *J Lab Clin Med* 1988;111(5):566–70.
18. Ascari E. Iron-deficiency anemia resistant to iron therapy. *Haematologica* 1993;78:178–82.
19. Cook JD, Lipschitz DA, Miles LE, Finch CA. Serum ferritin as a measure of iron stores in normal subjects. *Am J Clin Nutr* 1974;27(7):681–7.
20. Brolin RE, Gorman JH, Gorman RC, et al. Prophylactic iron supplementation after Roux-en-Y gastric bypass: A prospective, double-blind, randomized study. *Arch Surg* 1998;133:740–4.

# CHAPTER 13

# Zinc

Zinc is an essential trace mineral with literally hundreds of functions in the human body. There are perhaps 200 or more zinc-dependant enzymes that catalyze all manner of reactions in the body. These enzymes include those involved in acid-base reactions, digestion, cellular respiration, deoxyribonucleic acid (DNA) and ribonucleic acid (RNA) transcription, immune function, and antioxidant activity. In addition, zinc has nonenzymatic functions in growth and development, skin health, host defense/immunity, protein and cell membrane structure, and genetic transcription.

The overall absorption process for zinc is still not perfectly understood. It is not believed that the stomach plays much of a role in zinc digestion. Zinc absorption has not generally been demonstrated to be impaired in achlorhydria;[1] however, one study did show markedly reduced uptake from the digestive system in patients on omeprazole.[2] Zinc is known to be absorbed throughout the small intestine. Hydrolysis by proteases and nucleases frees dietary zinc from proteins. It is thought that most absorption occurs in the distal duodenum and proximal jejunum.[3] Absorption appears to be regulated by local levels of intestinal metallothionein. Overall, about 20 to 40 percent of ingested zinc is absorbed, although this may rise as high as 90 percent in acute depletion.

Zinc can be absorbed both through an active process at specialized binding sites or through passive diffusion. Some zinc is retained in local enterocytes and never goes into circulation. The remainder travels to the liver before being distributed to organs and tissues throughout the body. Most zinc is transported by albumen; the remainder is transported by ceruloplasmin, transferrin, and alpha-2-macroglobulin. Zinc is used by virtually every type of tissue in the body. The eyes, heart, adrenals, lungs, brain, skin, and prostate (in men) all store zinc. Adults store 2 to 3 grams of zinc; however, unlike most other minerals, zinc from tissues cannot be readily mobilized to compensate for low dietary intake.

Dietary factors can significantly impair or assist zinc absorption. Zinc is found in most animal proteins, including eggs (yolk) and dairy products. These tend to be the best sources as zinc is better absorbed in the presence of protein. Nuts, seeds, and whole grains are also substantial sources of zinc. However, phytates and fiber in grains may significantly impair absorption, making these sources less bioavailable. Refined grains, such as white rice, have very little zinc, as it is primarily found in the germ. The presence of unabsorbed dietary fat also diminishes zinc absorption, making fat malabsorption a risk for zinc deficiency. Other dietary elements that may impair zinc absorption include the presence of oxalate, polyphenols, and excess iron.

## DEFICIENCY

Zinc deficiency is still not well understood outside of the genetic form (acrodermatitis enteropathica). Deficiencies have been found with malabsorption, eating disorders, Crohn's disease, and Celiac disease. Serious injury, illness, stress, burns, and surgery increase zinc utilization and may contribute to deficiency. One problem that will be discussed later is that there are no highly sensitive or specific lab tests to determine zinc status.

Reported signs and symptoms of zinc deficiency can affect a wide variety of systems as zinc plays so many roles in the body. If dietary zinc intake is not adequate to fulfill needs, the body will free zinc from enzymes. Zinc is preferentially released from less critical systems and enzymes that bind it less tightly and is redistributed to more vital organs. Signs of chronic deficiency can include symptoms of loss of smell, abnormal or diminished sense of taste, poor wound healing, skin rashes or rough skin, hair loss/thinning hair, poor appetite, lethargy, grooved or deformed nails, decreased libido (men), canker sores, and more frequent infections. If deficiency progresses, an acquired form of acrodermatitis enteropathica can develop. Symptoms include loss of appetite or anorexia, diarrhea (which can be causative), photophobia, loss of night vision, significant hair loss (can be total), serious nail deformity, and a distinctly demarcated rash affecting the perioral, perianal, and genital areas. The rash can take a number of forms from eczematous to blistered to pustular. Significant inflammation or infection of the nail beds may be present. Behavioral and emotional symptoms similar to depression can also occur.

Zinc deficiency has been explored to a limited degree in both duodenal switch (DS) and Roux-en-y (RNY) weight loss surgeries. Several studies exploring changes in taste discrimination after RNY have found normal levels.[4,5]

A recent study published in *Obesity Surgery* compared preoperative zinc levels with two-month postoperative levels.[6] Researchers found that plasma and urinary levels fell while red blood cell (RBC) levels of zinc went from low to normal. Diet analysis done with the study showed that intake fell by an average of eight percent, although largely patients started out below the recommended daily allowance (RDA) and fell lower. Researchers concluded that based on these early labs and low intake, zinc deficiency likely could develop long-term.

Because hair loss can be experienced after weight loss surgery (WLS), the association between zinc and hair loss has drawn some interest. A group of researchers in England chose to study high dose zinc supplementation as a therapeutic agent for WLS-related hair loss.[7] The 1996 intervention trial administered 200mg of zinc sulfate (45mg elemental zinc) three times daily to postoperative patients with hair loss. This was in addition to the multivitamin and iron supplements that patients were already taking. No labs for zinc or other nutrients were conducted. Researchers found that in patients taking the zinc, 100 percent had cessation of hair loss after six months. In five patients, hair loss resumed after zinc was stopped and was arrested again with renewed supplementation. It is important to note that in telogen effluvium (diffuse hair loss) of non-nutritional origin, hair loss normally would be expected to stop within six months. In the absence of any laboratory studies, and with no placebo, the only patients of interest here are those who began to lose hair again after stopping zinc.

Clearly, longer studies are needed to truly understand zinc deficiency after RNY. With more malabsorptive procedures, zinc deficiency appears to be a common occurrence. Two separate studies have shown deficiency rates of 68 percent in biliopancreatic diversion (BPD) after one year and 50 percent (BPD and DS) after four years, respectively. These rates reflect impaired zinc absorption with fat malabsorption.

## LAB EVALUATION

As stated above, there is no highly sensitive or specific test for zinc deficiency. Plasma or serum zinc levels are the most common and have the best established reference ranges but have limitations that must be recognized. Levels should be obtained while the patient is fasting for greatest accuracy. Samples should not be allowed to sit longer than one hour and should be free of hemolysis. Plastic tubes should be avoided, and if testing plasma it is important to use a heparin tube (EDTA chelates zinc). If patients are sick, pregnant, using oral contraceptives or hormone replacement, or experiencing acute stress, levels may be altered. If patients are protein deficient, plasma zinc levels may be low in the absence of real deficiency due to albumen being the major carrier.

Intracellular levels of zinc are thought to be a more stable assessment of zinc status. White blood cell (WBC) levels are difficult to obtain but are thought to be more reflective of total body levels. RBC levels are available from national labs. They are thought to be a good assessment of chronic deficiency because of the 120-day lifespan of the erythrocyte.

Some zinc-dependent enzymes are measurable. The most readily available assay is plasma alkaline phosphatase (alk phos), but some studies have indicated that it does not always

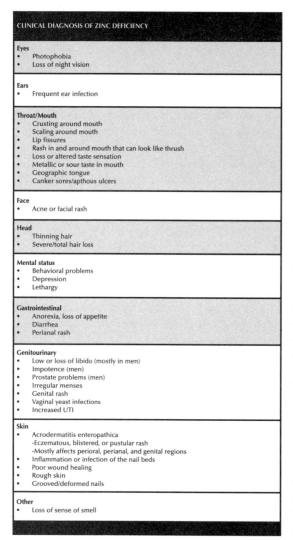

| CLINICAL DIAGNOSIS OF ZINC DEFICIENCY |
|---|
| **Eyes** |
| • Photophobia |
| • Loss of night vision |
| **Ears** |
| • Frequent ear infection |
| **Throat/Mouth** |
| • Crusting around mouth |
| • Scaling around mouth |
| • Lip fissures |
| • Rash in and around mouth that can look like thrush |
| • Loss or altered taste sensation |
| • Metallic or sour taste in mouth |
| • Geographic tongue |
| • Canker sores/apthous ulcers |
| **Face** |
| • Acne or facial rash |
| **Head** |
| • Thinning hair |
| • Severe/total hair loss |
| **Mental status** |
| • Behavioral problems |
| • Depression |
| • Lethargy |
| **Gastrointestinal** |
| • Anorexia, loss of appetite |
| • Diarrhea |
| • Perianal rash |
| **Genitourinary** |
| • Low or loss of libido (mostly in men) |
| • Impotence (men) |
| • Prostate problems (men) |
| • Irregular menses |
| • Genital rash |
| • Vaginal yeast infections |
| • Increased UTI |
| **Skin** |
| • Acrodermatitis enteropathica |
|   -Eczematous, blistered, or pustular rash |
|   -Mostly affects perioral, perianal, and genital regions |
| • Inflammation or infection of the nail beds |
| • Poor wound healing |
| • Rough skin |
| • Grooved/deformed nails |
| **Other** |
| • Loss of sense of smell |

change with low zinc. Levels appear to rise in response to treatment in deficiency established by other methods.[8] Thus alk phos levels may be useful for tracking response to treatment. Plasma 5-nucleotidease levels are more sensitive, but are not readily available. Angiotensin converting enzyme (ACE) is zinc-dependent, but does not appear to useful in humans. There is some availability of RBC metallothionein, which appears to be a stable assessment of long-term zinc status.

Zinc assessments in hair are available but are not considered to be standardized or accurate. Urine levels will fall in response to low intake as the body tries to prevent loss. Testosterone levels can be low with zinc deficiency, and this may be an incidental finding in men reporting infertility, low libido, or sexual dysfunction. It is worth noting here that there is an older case report in a jejunoileal bypass (JIB) patient reporting with fatigue, weakness, low libido, and impotence.[9] His diagnosis included zinc deficiency and subsequent low testosterone.

## TREATMENT

For mild zinc deficiency, doses of 15 to 30 milligrams per day taken between meals and away from other minerals should be tried. It is best to leave two hours between zinc supplements and iron- or copper-containing supplements. If patients also have low calcium, zinc and calcium should be taken separately as high-dose zinc supplements may further impair calcium absorption. Zinc often causes digestive irritation, much like iron, so initiating therapy at this level is more gentle and may be all that is required. In more severe deficiency, higher doses in the range of 30 to 150mg may be required for weeks to months for symptoms to resolve. These should be given in divided doses, and clinicians should watch for side effects, such as diarrhea, that may make therapy nonproductive. If digestive upset is persistent, patients can take zinc with a protein drink or protein food. This may actually assist absorption somewhat.

There are many preparations of zinc supplements available. The most common forms are sulfate and gluconate. One can also find other amino acid–bound forms as well as other chelates. These forms may be better absorbed and better tolerated. Clinicians should note that like iron, zinc preparations may come labeled with either the dose of the total compound or the elemental dose. The elemental amount of the mineral varies by preparation and it needs to be known as that is on what recommendations are based. Patients taking doses in excess of 30mg/day should do so in divided doses. Some percentage of patients may still report gastrointestinal (GI) distress at this level, and smaller increments may need to be given. Zinc lozenges, often sold in the cold care section of the pharmacy, can be a great choice for WLS patients who cannot swallow pills. The labels should be read for sugar content, but sugar-free preparations are available. Zinc nasal solutions have not been evaluated as systemic supplements and are not advised. Zinc chloride and sulfate are both available for injection. Exact dosing for injection is not known. Estimates are made at around 2 to 4mg for an adult.

In addition to monitoring plasma zinc and symptoms for recovery, patients should be monitored for copper deficiency, which can develop as a side effect. Assuring that patients are at least taking a multivitamin with 1 to 3mg of zinc is a good protective strategy.

## PREVENTION AND MAINTENANCE

The RDA for zinc is 15mg for men and 12mg for women. This level is commonly found in a multivitamin. Amino acid–bound forms like zinc methionine and chelates like zinc gluconate or citrate are more gentle on the digestive system and may be better absorbed. Until more is known, it would be wise for RNY patients to take a multivitamin with the RDA for zinc.

We do not know the levels of zinc needed to prevent deficiency in any type of WLS. BPD/DS patients taking the levels in a multivitamin still developed significant deficiencies of zinc. Since the likely cause of this is steatorrhoea, having patients take zinc supplements on an empty stomach or with a low-fat/fat-free, protein-based meal may overcome some of the problem. As noted above, taking zinc with protein or protein supplements may even benefit absorption to a degree. For prevention, a dose of 15 to 30mg once daily can be tried. Unfortunately, this can be challenging for adherence. Sometimes, asking patients to take this dose first thing in the morning or at bedtime can improve conformity.

Zinc in the diet is readily obtained from shellfish, other seafood, meat, dairy products, eggs, legumes, nuts, and seeds.

## EXCESS AND TOXICITY

As with iron, therapeutic levels of zinc overlap with toxic levels, so it is important to know what can occur. Acute toxicity of zinc most commonly presents with gastrointestinal upset. The most common symptoms are abdominal pain, diarrhea, nausea, vomiting, and metallic taste in the mouth. This can happen at doses as low as 30mg, but is more common with doses exceeding 100mg. If using these levels for therapy, divided doses usually reduce or eliminate the problems in the gut. Chronic toxicity from excess long-term use can occur at doses as low as 60 total milligrams from combined food and supplemental sources. The most common sign of chronic overload is copper deficiency (zinc competes with copper). Copper deficiency presents as a microcytic, hypochromic anemia that is unresponsive to iron therapy. There also may be low white cell counts, fever, chills, and mouth sores. Much more rare are skin and neurological problems. High-density lipoprotein (HDL) levels can also drop in individuals on zinc therapy.[10] Additionally worth noting is the recent AREDS study (Age-Related Eye Disease Study) that utilized 80mg of zinc as zinc oxide in one protocol. In the high-dose zinc group, about 7.5 percent of participants had urinary tract problems that required hospitalization. Thus, we should consider urinary tract infections, kidney stones, incontinence, and enlarged prostate as possible signs of zinc overload.

## INTERACTIONS

Use of zinc with quinolones, tetracyclines, and bisphosphonates can decrease levels of both drug and nutrient. Zinc should not be taken with testosterone or other androgen-elevating drugs unless under physician supervision as these drugs may cause abnormal elevations of zinc. Some anticoagulants like warfarin can complex with zinc in the gut, so they should be taken two hours apart. Calcium, copper, and iron can all interact with zinc, and concomitant use should likely be avoided in patients treating deficiencies or requiring high doses of any of these minerals.

## CONCLUSION

There are probably more deficiencies of zinc after WLS than are reported in literature. Patients such as those with DS procedures should be monitored regularly with lab studies and made familiar with common symptoms so they can report problems. We do not know whether regular monitoring would be of any value in RNY. Clinicians should be aware of the potential risks and symptoms of deficiency. Assuring adequate intake through diet and a multivitamin is good advice in RNY until more is known.

## REFERENCES

1.    Andstrom B, Abrahamsson H. Zinc absorption and achlorhydria. *Eur J Clin Nutr* 1989 Dec;43(12):877–9.
2.    Ozutemiz AO, Aydin HH, Isler M, et al. Effect of omeprazole on plasma zinc levels after oral zinc administration. *Indian J Gastroenterol* 2002;21(6):216–8.
3.    Krebs NF, Westcott JE, Huffer JW, Miller LV. Absorption of exogenous zinc and secretion of endogenous zinc in the human small intestine. *FASEB J* 1998;12:A345.
4.    Scruggs DM, Buffington C, Cowan GS Jr. Taste acuity of the morbidly obese before and after gastric bypass surgery. *Obes Surg* 1994;4(1):24–8.
5.    Burge JC, Schaumburg JZ, Choban PS, et al. Changes in patients' taste acuity after Roux-en-Y gastric bypass for clinically severe obesity. *J Am Diet Assoc* 1995;95(6):666–70.
6.    Cominetti C, Garrido AB, Cozzolino SMF. Zinc nutritional status of morbidly obese patients before and after Roux-en-Y bypass: A preliminary report. *Obes Surg* 2006;16(4):448–53.
7.    Neve H, Bhatti W, Soulsby C, et al. Reversal of hair loss following vertical gastroplasty when treated with zinc sulphate. *Obes Surg* 1996;6(1):63–5.
8.    Kasarskis EJ, Schuna A. Serum alkaline phosphatase after treatment of zinc deficiency in humans. *Am J Clin Nutr* 1980;33(12):2609–12.
9.    Schuetz P, Peterli R, Ludwid C, Peters T. Fatigue,weakness, and sexual dysfunction after bariatric surgery: Not an unusual case but an unusual cause. *Obes Surg* 2004;14(7):1025–8.
10.   Hooper R, Laurent V, Garry P. Zinc lowers high-density lipoprotein cholesterol levels. *JAMA* 1980;244(17):1960–1.

# CHAPTER 14

# Copper

Copper is an essential trace element that is a small but important player in human nutrition. Copper plays varied roles in the body in antioxidant nutrition, energy production, connective tissue health, nervous system health, neurotransmitter and melanin production, and regulation of gene expression.

Acquired copper deficiency is thought to be quite rare, occurring only in association with discrete medical conditions. Conditions known to contribute to copper deficiency are prolonged infection or inflammation, pregnancy, liver disease, use of estrogenic drugs, celiac disease, surgical resection of the bowel, nephritic syndrome, and generalized

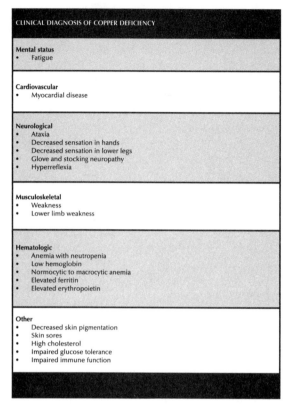

malnutrition. Cases are also reported with long-term use of total enteral or parenteral nutrition, as well as with excessive or prolonged intake of iron[1] or zinc[2] supplements.

## LAB FINDINGS

Hematological disorder is thought to be the major manifestation of adult acquired copper deficiency. Interestingly, it is associated with more than one presentation of anemia. The combined presentation of anemia and neutropenia appears to be a hallmark of copper deficiency. In isolated copper deficiency, other findings appear to include somewhat low to low-normal hemoglobin, normocytic or mildly macrocytic anemia (elevated mean corpuscular volume [MCV]), and normal platelet counts.[3] Elevated ferritin and erythropoietin (EPO) may also be seen. These findings are similar to those seen in Menkes disease (an inherited disorder of copper metabolism). Ceruloplasmin, an enzyme and carrier protein containing eight copper atoms, can also be measured and is low with copper deficiency.

It is not uncommon to see literature indicating that microcytic hypochromic anemia is the finding in copper deficiency. Healthy copper status is required for normal iron transport. It appears that when copper is depleted, iron is not properly transported from storage to the bone marrow for production of red blood cells.[4] This might explain the finding of elevated ferritin in some cases of copper deficiency. Chronic copper deficiency could therefore result in disordered iron metabolism and an anemia that mimics that of iron deficiency. In these cases, serum iron and ferritin should still be normal, and neutropenia would still be expected. In the case of weight loss surgery (WLS), however, it might be possible to see true combined deficiency since both nutrients can be malabsorbed. If this were the case, neutropenia might be the only distinct hematological feature. Copper deficiency might become more suspect if anemia did not correct as expected with iron therapy or in any way worsened with iron therapy.

## OTHER FINDINGS

The Mayo Clinic recently reported on four cases of copper deficiency in adults that manifested with the primary condition of myelopathy.[5] Two of the reported cases were in gastric surgery: One after a Billroth II procedure for an ulcer and the other after gastric bypass. While the anemia of copper deficiency has been recognized for a long time, copper deficiency leading to myelopathy was only first described in 2001 in a single case report.[6] Since that time, perhaps 15 to 30 other cases have been identified, mostly in association with zinc excess. Patients described by the doctors at the Mayo Clinic presented with mild anemia that had been presumed to be due to iron deficiency. They then manifested ataxia, decreased sensation in the hands and lower legs, lower limb weakness, and hyper-reflexia. Magnetic resonance imaging (MRI) studies done in other cases has revealed subacute combined degeneration very similar to that seen in B12 deficiency, which would explain the similar symptoms.

Other possible signs of deficiency include generalized weakness and fatigue, decreased skin pigmentation, skin wounds, increased cholesterol, poor immune function, impaired glucose tolerance, and myocardial disease. There are also rare case reports of apparent copper-induced pancytopenia and sideroblastic anemia.

## ABSORPTION AND METABOLISM

Studies of copper absorption in patients with Wilson's disease have demonstrated that maximal absorption occurs in the proximal gut. Small amounts may also be absorbed directly from the stomach itself. The overall amount of copper absorbed as a percentage of the dose can vary significantly, but averages about 30 to 40 percent. There is significant competition between copper absorption and both iron and zinc. High supplementation of either nutrient, especially if dietary copper intake was low, could easily contribute to inducing deficiency.[7] Much like iron, copper relies on stomach acid to free it from its bound state in food and to help maintain the optimal ionic state for absorption. Thus it can be expected that procedures like gastric bypass surgery create a barrier to copper absorption. Copper status could further be hampered in WLS patients by the commonly recommended doses of iron and in some cases by zinc supplementation.

Once absorbed, copper is transported to the liver by albumen. For this reason, it is possible that a low protein intake could adversely affect copper metabolism. Once in the liver, it is incorporated into ceruloplasmin and various enzyme systems and bile.

## DISCUSSION

Both anemia and neuropathy are common nutritional complications of WLS. There are numerous case reports in literature of cases where anemia and neuropathy cannot be linked to a clear cause. The authors of the Mayo study point out that copper studies have generally not been included in the differential diagnosis of these cases. Based on these findings, copper deficiency should likely be considered before other presumptive diagnoses are made. Copper deficiency should also be considered in anemia that does not correct or that worsens with iron supplementation, and any case of combined anemia with neutropenia.

Nutritional textbooks often list the measurement of copper-zinc superoxide dismutase activity as the best indication of long-term status. However, this test may not be readily available and may be quite expensive when it is. Measurements of serum copper or ceruloplasmin are generally available and are adequate indicators of status.

The dietary reference intake (DRI) for copper is 900mcg. The Institute of Medicine has set the tolerable upper limit (UL) at 10mg (10,000mcg) per day. Doses of 3 to 5mg of copper have often been recommended to correct deficiency. It is not known whether this would be adequate in WLS patients, but as it is well under the UL it is clearly safe. If deficient patients are also supplementing iron and/or zinc, care should be given to have patients take these supplements at separate times. It has been suggested that 1mg of copper should be supplemented for each 8 to 15mg of zinc. While high levels of iron are known to interfere with copper absorption, an ideal ratio is not known.

Copper supplements come in a variety of forms. Copper sulfate, citrate, and gluconate are all relatively common. The citrate and gluconate forms are generally easier on the digestive system, and may be preferred in WLS patients. Good dietary sources for copper include organ meats, shellfish, nuts, beans/legumes, dark chocolate, enriched grains, dried fruits, mushrooms, tomatoes, potatoes, bananas, grapes, and avocados.

Cases such as those reported by Mayo indicate that we still have much to learn about general human nutrition, and even more so about nutrition and WLS. It is likely that more cases of copper deficiency exist among current WLS patients, and more will be reported in the future.

## REFERENCES

1.    Yadrick MK, Kenney MA, Winterfeldt EA. Iron, copper, and zinc status: Response to supplementation with zinc or zinc and iron in adult females. *Am J Clin Nutr* 1989;49(1):145–50.
2.    Fosmire GJ. Zinc toxicity. *Am J Clin Nutr* 1990;51(2):225–7.
3.    Uauy R, Olivares M, Gonzalez M. Essentiality of copper in humans. *Am J Clin Nutr* 1998;67(5 Suppl):952S–9S.
4.    Kumar N, Ahlskog JE, Gross JB Jr. Acquired hypocupremia after gastric surgery. *Clin Gastroenterol Hepatol* 2004;2(12):1074–9.
5.    Schleper B, Stuerenburg HJ. Copper deficiency-associated myelopathy in a 46-year-old woman. *J Neurol* 2001;248:705–6.
6.    Yadrick MK, Kenney MA, Winterfeldt EA. Iron, copper, and zinc status: Response to supplementation with zinc or zinc and iron in adult females. *Am J Clin Nutr* 1989;49(1):145–50.

# CHAPTER 15

# Selenium

S elenium is a trace element that is essential to the formation of selenoproteins in the body. In humans, most selenoproteins are antioxidant enzymes, including the four glutathione peroxidases and thioredoxin reductase. It is for this reason that selenium is sometimes classified as an antioxidant and frequently appears in antioxidant dietary supplements. Three separate selenoproteins act as thyroid hormone deiodinases. Deiodination is necessary to both the activation and inactivation of thyroid hormones. As thyroid hormones are important to growth, development, and metabolism, selenium is critical to these processes. Both selenium deficiency and excess result in diminished

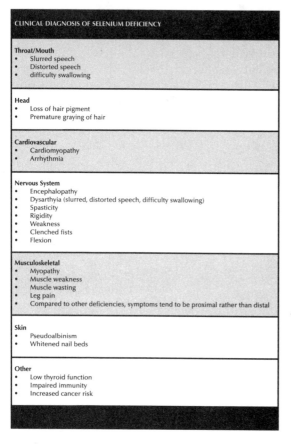

thyroid activity. Other selenoproteins function in protein transport, muscle metabolism, and the synthesis of selenoproteins themselves. Outside of the its role in the selenoproteins, selenium may be important to immune function, detoxification (especially of heavy metals), deoxyribonucleic acid (DNA) repair, and induction of the cytochrome P450 system.

Selenium has garnered recent attention for its potential role in cancer prevention. Several large studies have examined selenium intake and cancer risk and have shown an association with rates of occurrence for specific cancers. These studies include a 1996 report published in the *Journal of the American Medical Association* that found that selenium at three times the current recommended daily allowance (RDA) led to 63-percent fewer cases of prostate cancer, 58-percent fewer cases of rectal cancer, 47-percent fewer cases of lung cancer, and an overall 50-percent reduction in total cancer deaths.[1] Numerous studies have since demonstrated similar results. Based on the totality of these findings, the US Food and Drug Administration (FDA) recently allowed a qualified health claim for selenium and cancer prevention[2]—a rarity for the FDA for any nutrient.

Selenium in the diet comes in two primary forms: Selenoproteins that occur naturally in plant and animal products and sodium selenite that is fed to animals in areas with selenium-poor soil or is found in some dietary supplements. Sodium selenite is also used in nutritional products. Selenium is generally well absorbed, although it is believed that selenomethionine is the best absorbed form. Selenomethionine has been demonstrated to be up to 90-percent bioavailable in studies of absorption.[3] Most uptake occurs in the duodenum; some uptakes can occur in the jejunum and ileum. Absorption appears to be enhanced by the presence of other antioxidants like vitamins E and C. Mercury and other heavy metals inhibit absorption.

Once absorbed, selenium is transported by low-density lipoproteins (LDL) and very low-density lipoproteins (VLDL). It is then incorporated into the selenoproteins by a process that is not fully understood. Selenium can be stored in selenoproteins and muscle, as well as in some organs, such as the liver, kidney, and pancreas. The body stores about 15mg of selenium in total.

## DEFICIENCY

Selenium deficiency is thought to be rare in the general population. The mineral is widespread in animal products, especially organ meats and seafood. Plant products contain varying amounts of selenium depending on where they are grown. This is because plants do not require selenium, but will absorb it from soil if it is present. Before animal feeds were selenium-enriched, the amount of selenium in meats varied much more depending on from where the meat came. Most feeds now contain selenium, which largely makes up for regional variability.

Gastrointestinal surgery has been documented as a cause of selenium deficiency, but deficiency is primarily seen in people with Crohn's disease.[4] A 1988 study examined selenium and zinc status in jejunoileal bypass (JIB) surgery patients and found significantly reduced selenium status,[5] but we cannot necessarily correlate this to modern procedures. The reality is that selenium status is largely undocumented, so we cannot make an informed statement about possible incidence. Still, based on where the majority of selenium is absorbed, it can be considered to be a risk.

As deficiency is uncommon, a typical clinical presentation has not been established. In areas where there is selenium-poor soil and people are largely restricted to local food sources, there are endemic conditions related to selenium deficiency. Keshan and Kashin-Beck disease occur primarily in rural parts of Asia and affect the heart and the connective tissue, respectively. Keshan disease is actually thought to be a viral condition to which selenium deficiency creates susceptibility, whereas Kashin-Beck disease appears to be due to the combined influences of selenium and iodine deficiency with environmental factors. The most clear picture we have of selenium deficiency comes from its symptoms that arise from total parenteral nutrition (TPN).[6] These symptoms include myopathy, cardiomyopathy, arrhythmia, and muscle wasting. Muscle weakness and pain is more commonly reported in the legs and is more proximal than distal. Symptoms can also include impaired immunity, low thyroid function, loss of skin and hair pigmentation, and whitened nail beds.[7] Severe loss of skin pigmentation has been reported in case reports, manifesting as pseudoalbinism.[8] Progressive encephalopathy has also been reported.[9] There are also sporadic case reports of encephalopathy in children with selenium deficiency due to TPN. Reported symptoms include dysarthria (slurred, distorted speech, difficulty swallowing), spasticity, weakness, rigidity, clenched fists, and flexion (decorticate posturing).

## LAB EVALUATION

Plasma and serum selenium concentrations are only reflective of recent intake and tell little about long-term or functional status. Selenium levels can also be measured in red blood cells (RBCs), which would reflect a three-month period. For functional assessment, measurement of glutathione peroxidase activity is the best accepted method. This can be assessed in platelets, RBCs, or plasma. RBC levels have the longest half-life and are probably the preferred medium. Platelet levels are also well accepted.

Hair and toenail clippings also are often used to assess selenium status. There appears to be a good correlation between these levels and tissue levels. Hair minerals, however, are greatly affected by exposure to the environment, and there is data indicating that laboratory methods for evaluating hair samples are poorly standardized and unreliable.[10] Samples of toenails likely reflect selenium levels 6 to 9 months in the past, and so are not good measures of current status. Additionally, the test is not readily available.

Other lab studies that show low thyroid hormones, high thyroid stimulating hormone (TSH), low vitamin E, elevated homocysteine,[11] increased mean corpuscular volume (MCV) (macrocytosis),[12] and elevated creatinine kinase levels are also indicative of selenium deficiency.

## TREATMENT

Because selenium is well absorbed outside the duodenum, oral supplementation should be adequate for most cases of deficiency. A typical therapeutic dose is 200mcg/day. Refractory cases may require intravenous (IV) replacement. Doses of 40 to 100mcg can be given daily for up to a month if needed. Often this is done in combination with other trace elements like copper, zinc, chromium, and manganese. It may be beneficial to supplement vitamins E, C, and A with selenium as they appear to help uptake. By either route of administration, improvements are usually significant at four weeks.

## PREVENTION AND MAINTENANCE

There is no data to indicate what levels of selenium are needed after any kind of WLS. The RDA for selenium is 55mcg and the daily value (DV) is 70mcg. Most multivitamins provide between 60 and 120mcg. Selenium-rich foods include Brazil nuts, seafood (especially shell fish), meat, milk, and brown rice.

## EXCESS AND TOXICITY

Selenium, like most trace elements, can be toxic if too much is taken. The Institute of Medicine sets 400mcg as the tolerable upper limit (UL) based on the ability of chronic toxicity to develop at that level. Acute toxicity has been reported with accidental ingestion of levels far above that (over 27,000mcg), levels that should be impossible under any normal circumstance. Early signs of toxicity are nail breakage, hair breakage and loss, and fatigue. Later signs may include rashes, loss of hair and nails, nausea, vomiting, and neurological disturbances. It is worth noting that healthy men fed diets with approximately 300mcg of selenium developed clinical hypothyroidism and weight gain after only 99 days.[13]

## INTERACTIONS
Selenium may reduce the effectiveness of some chemotherapeutic agents, especially bleomycin. Thus, it should not be combined with these treatments unless advised. Cigarette smoking reduces selenium levels in the body, meaning that smokers may require more. It is possible that high doses of iron or zinc may reduce absorption of selenium from food or dietary supplements.

## CONCLUSION

Selenium is a trace mineral about which there is not much information available in regards to the WLS patient. Current data tells us nothing about occurrence of deficiency. It could be a risk based on knowledge of other procedures leading to deficiency. Levels in diet and in multivitamins should be adequate to maintain normal levels in most individuals, but clinicians should be aware of what can occur with deficiency. It is unlikely that regular screening will ever be advised as deficiency is generally so rare; however, tests should be ordered if symptoms are present and other more likely causes are ruled out. Other more commonly deficient nutrients that could cause similar symptoms include thiamine and B12.

## REFERENCES

1.  Clark L, Combs GF, Turnbull BW, et al. Effects of selenium supplementation for cancer prevention in patients with carcinoma of the skin. *JAMA* 1996;276(24):1957–63.
2.  Allowable claim per FDA letter dated February 11, 2003:"Selenium may reduce the risk of certain cancers. Some scientific evidence suggests that consumption of selenium may reduce the risk of certain forms of cancer. However, FDA has determined that this evidence is limited and not conclusive."
3.  Food and Nutrition Board, Institute of Medicine. Selenium. *Dietary reference intakes for vitamin C, vitamin E, selenium, and carotenoids.* Washington DC: National Academy Press, 2000:284–324.
4.  Rannem T, Ladefoged K, Hylander E, et al. Selenium status in patients with Crohn's disease. *Am J Clin Nutr* 1992;56(5):933–7.
5.  Gjorup I, Gjorup T, Andersen B. Serum selenium and zinc concentrations in morbid obesity. Comparison of controls and patients with jejunoileal bypass. *Scand J Gastroenterol* 1988;23(10):1250–2.
6.  Gramm HJ, Kopf A, Bratter P. The necessity of selenium substitution in total parenteral nutrition and artificial alimentation. *J Trace Elem Med Biol* 1995;9(1):1–12.
7.  Nakamura N, Nokura K. Selenium deficiency in a patient with Crohn's disease receiving long-term total parenteral nutrition. *Internal Medicine* 2003;42:154–7.
8.  Vinton NE, Dahlstrom KA, Strobel CT, Ament ME. Macrocytosis and pseudoalbinism: Manifestations of selenium deficiency. *J Pediatr* 1987;111(5):711–7.
9.  Kawakubo K, Iida M, Matsumoto T, et al. Progressive encephalopathy in a Crohn's disease patient on long-term total parenteral nutrition: Possible relationship to selenium deficiency. *Postgrad Med J* 1994;70(821):215–9.
10. Seidel S, Kreutzer R, Smith D, et al. Assessment of commercial laboratories performing hair mineral analysis. *JAMA* 2001;285:67–72.
11. Gonzalez S, Huerta JM, Alvarez-Uria J, et al. Serum selenium is associated with plasma homocysteine concentrations in elderly humans. *J Nutr* 2004;134(7):1736–40.
12. Vinton NE, Dahlstrom KA, Strobel CT, Ament ME. Macrocytosis and pseudoalbinism: Manifestations of selenium deficiency. *J Pediatr* 1987;111(5):711–7.
13. Hawkes WC, Keim NL. Dietary selenium intake modulates thyroid hormone and energy metabolism in men. *J Nutr* 2003;133(11):3443–8.

# PART 3: Putting It All Together—Strategies for Risk Reduction

When we look at the big picture of weight loss surgery (WLS) and nutrition, prevention should be the focus over treatment. One challenge that clearly faces those caring for post-WLS patients—at least as of the writing of this book— is that there is no accepted standard of care. To be fair, based on the current data we have, the best that can be said with total assurance of clinical and scientific accuracy is:

1. WLS creates nutritional risk.
2. Preventive nutrition through diet and supplementation is important.
3. Regular follow up and nutritional assessment is important and should be lifelong.
4. Patient education that stresses adherence is an important component of nutritional health.

Truthfully, we do not yet have enough data to tell us exactly when levels of nutrients will clearly prevent the development of common deficiencies in patients. Given all the variables in human nutrition and the fact that we still cannot clearly define preventive nutrition levels for people who have not had WLS, we may be looking at years before clear recommendations exist. The focus, then, should rightly be on risk reduction. It is much easier to answer the question: How do we lower the risk of nutritional problems in WLS patients? than to answer: How do we prevent nutritional problems from developing?

## HAVE A CLEAR PLAN

Patients are much more likely to adopt and adhere to a nutrition program that is clearly defined for them. In the absence of a clear plan, it is much easier for patients to adopt the latest fad they have read about on the internet or the advice that they have received from well-meaning friends or do nothing at all. Because dietary supplements vary in form, quality, and potency, it is best for a program to prescreen and select dietary supplements for the patients. This helps the patients because they will not get distracted by the sea of products at their local nutrition store; it also helps the practitioner (you) because if something does go wrong, you know exactly what your patients are taking. For more on selecting products to use in your practice, please see Appendix B in the back of the book. Patients also tend to adhere to specific recommendations better than vague ones. For example, you will get better adherence if you say, "I want you to go to the pharmacy and get Brand X chewable calcium and take two per day," versus saying, "I want you take calcium supplements." You will also get fewer calls to your office from patients who are in the store trying to select one of two dozen brands.

## EDUCATION AND FOLLOW-UP

Education is an incredibly important part of nutritional counseling. If patients understand not only what you are asking them to do but also why it is important to do it and what the expectations are, they are more likely to adhere to the treatment. When it comes to nutrition, most patients need to hear it regularly. If they are only told preoperatively and/or in the immediate postoperative period, they will forget.

In their 1991 study, Georgeann Mallory and Alex MacGregor concluded the following: "We attribute the low incidence of folate deficiency found in our postoperative patient population compared with previous reports to a strong follow-up program. These patients are subjected to a continual barrage of exhortation to maintain their multivitamin supplements. Simply put, in a bariatric surgical practice in which patients are encouraged, reminded, and even badgered into taking postoperative supplements, the occurrence of folate deficiency should be a rarity."

Adherence is always higher with regular reminders and support groups, and scheduled visits bring patients back. This is critical for all-around nutritional success in both maintaining good eating habits and supplement use.

The things that people say when they call my office often astonish me. One regular statement I hear is that patients feel they have been told that they only need to supplement for one or two years after surgery. When I ask them why, they often say, "Well they didn't ask to see me back after that so I thought I was done." Clear communication in regards to nutritional expectation needs to be both set and reinforced. For many nutrients, the incidence of deficiency continues to increase with the number of years one is out from surgery. Nutrition is a life-long commitment, not a temporary state.

With nutrition, you often have to fight what I call the "feel good phenomenon." When people feel good, nutrition is the first habit they neglect. This is where the idea of risk reduction needs to be implement, enforcing that the best time for good nutrition is when patients feel good because chances are it will help to keep them feeling good.

I try to explain this to patients by making a parallel to a drug therapy. Many patients have been on medications for high blood pressure or diabetes. I ask the following: "You would not stop taking your medication when your blood pressure or blood sugar became normal and you felt good, right? It is exactly the same for nutrition after WLS. If you stop taking your nutrition seriously, it is much more likely that something will go wrong that could really hurt your health."

People tend to get the analogy. Also consider writing a real prescription. I know that might sound silly, but it helps to put dietary supplements on a more equal par with a drug therapy for some patients. Nutrition is generally not taken seriously in our culture. Just as a white coat can transform the image of a person into a health professional, so too can a prescription pad transform an ordinary vitamin into a drug.

## BRINGING THEM BACK

Even among those with the best intentions, many people will fall off the bandwagon at some point in time. It is important for programs to have ways to try to stay in contact with patients and bring them back for their necessary follow-up, especially for things like annual lab testing. There are great computer programs that send e-mail reminders and there is always the old-fashioned phone call—many methods are available. In my office, we used to use post cards: Patients would write their own name and address and the office manager would file them in a special file for the week/month/year the next visit was to take place. Each week, she would go to the file and send out the cards. If any came back to our office, we knew that was a patient we needed to find.

Offering programs just for patients who need to get "back on track" is also a great way to keep patients in follow-up past the 1- to 2-year mark. This is especially great for patients who have slipped a bit. These patients do not feel comfortable coming to a group of excited, recent postoperatives who are losing weight rapidly and doing everything by the book.

## WHEN PATIENTS MOVE ON

Maybe your program is not equipped to manage patients long-term. Maybe you have patients who come from a large geographic area and cannot easily get to your office. Maybe you find, as your program matures, that patients move away or no longer want to come back to a bariatric program. Patients move on for many reasons, but it is still important for them to get the care they need. I strongly recommend having a set of instructions that patients can take with them to their primary care doctors. This may have a few words about the procedure, medications to avoid, cautions and warning signs of serious problems, recommended lab screens, and your contact information so they can call if needed. Because life-long care is essential, helping to create this continuity is in everyone's best interests.

# BASIC NUTRITION PROTOCOLS BY PROCEDURE

Because known levels of preventive nutrition are not established for WLS patients, these suggestions for risk reduction are very simple. I am a fan of not going overboard. More nutrition does not necessarily do more and may lose a larger number of patients to nonadherence. In some cases, such as supplementing high doses of iron prophylactically, there is the potential to do inadvertent harm.

## ADJUSTABLE GASTRIC BANDING (AGB)

Many programs recommend no nutrition after gastric banding. Generally after AGB, it is caloric restriction that produces weight loss. With caloric restriction there is reduced nutritional opportunity, and thus less of a chance that patients will meet nutritional needs through diet alone. Additionally, there is some evidence of nutritional deficiencies of thiamine, B12, and folate and loss of bone mass in patients who have undergone AGB. Based on these issues, it is advisable that some basic nutrition be recommended for AGB patients to help augment diet and reduce risk of any possible deficiencies.

### AGB General Recommendations
- Chewable multivitamin with B12 and iron (liquid or powder are also an option)
- Soft foods can be initiated usually Week 2 postoperative.
- When patients are comfortably eating regular foods, they can switch to smaller tablets or capsules of supplements if desired.
- Additional B12 and folate should be considered for the first two years. This may be simply accomplished by selecting a multivitamin that provides 800mcg folate and 50mcg or more of B12.
- A separate supplement of calcium should be considered. Providing an additional 500 to 1000mg of calcium per day can help to decrease the risk of bone loss. Assuring that vitamin D intake is adequate (from diet or multivitamin) is also important.

## ROUX-EN-Y GASTRIC BYPASS SURGERY (RNY)
It is generally well recognized that patients who have undergone RNY will require nutritional supplements to make up for both reduced food intake and malabsorption. Products for RNY patients should be carefully selected for bioavailability, quality, and nutrient content.

### RNY General Recommendations
- Chewable multivitamin starting from the first day patients return home from the hospital. (liquid or powder are also an option)
- Sublingual B12 (alternately, intranasal or injections)
- Iron at the level of the RDA for nonanemic patients. Iron may not need to be initiated immediately if patients are not anemic. Since iron can act as a direct GI irritant, patients should get through the first month after surgery, when there is the most digestive adjustment, without introducing iron. Start with a chewable or liquid. Patients can progress to a tablet or capsule after 3 to 6 months. The other option with iron is watchful waiting. This

has to be a clinical choice and may vary by patient (i.e., you might treat a young menstruating woman differently than a 40-year-old man or a patient who has adherence problems). Vitamin C has been shown to benefit iron absorption after RNY. Some products combine the two nutrients together. Vitamin C can also be added as a separate supplement if desired.

- One thousand to 1500 mg of calcium from calcium citrate is a good risk reduction strategy. It is best to advise that this be taken in divided doses of no more than 500mg at one time, and that it be taken away from iron dosing if iron is recommended. Patients can start calcium as a chewable, liquid, or powder when they are home from the hospital. Some patients experience gastrointestinal (GI) side effects from calcium. If this occurs, these patients should wait one month postoperatively before continuing with calcium.
- After 3 to 6 months, patients can usually switch to small tablets or capsulated supplements if they desire. Some find that chewable products remain the better option due to the number of pills or difficulty with swallowed forms.
- Some programs are now recommending additional thiamin in the first few months post-operatively. This sometimes comes as a recommendation to take a B-complex. My feeling is that this is best accomplished through a multivitamin, unless a patient needs the additional thiamin for therapeutic purposes.
- Nutrition must be lifelong. Patients need to commit to regular laboratory evaluations, and adjustments to the basic nutritional program may need to be made over time if problems arise.

## DUODENAL SWITCH (DS)

DS patients have greater malabsorption, especially of fat-soluble vitamins. For this reason, it is usually recommended that higher levels of A, E, D, and K be given proactively. Some programs also advise higher levels of calcium, zinc, and iron. There is much less data and less agreement on risk-reduction strategies for these patients.

### DS Recommendations
- Chewable multivitamin starting from the first day patients return home from the hospital. (liquid or powder are also an option)
- B12 in the range of 50 to 350mcg/day. This may be accomplished in the multivitamin. Some programs recommend higher levels akin to RNY.
- One thousand five hundred to 2000mg of calcium from calcium citrate is a good risk reduction strategy. It is best to advise that this be taken in divided doses of no more than 500mg at one and that it be taken away from iron dosing if iron is recommended. Patients can start calcium as a chewable, liquid, or powder when they are home from the hospital. Some patients experience gastrointestinal (GI) side effects from calcium. If this occurs, these patients should wait one month postoperatively before continuing with calcium.
- There is really no agreement on iron supplementation after DS. The range is watchful waiting (with no iron supplementation) up to 300mg of elemental iron/day. Clinicians are currently basing these choices on clinical experience. The tolerable upper limit (UL) for iron is 45mg, so dosing above this clearly has increased risks of negative effects in nonanemic patients.

While there is not enough data to properly advise, a range between the RDA and the UL is safe. Many iron supplements contain 45 to 55mg of elemental iron, just above the UL, which is probably within reason.

- Vitamin A as preformed retinol or dry vitamin A at levels of 10,000 to 30,000IU/day. Women who can get pregnant should be advised that these levels are considered to be potentially harmful, at least in women without malabsorption.
- Vitamin E as natural vitamin E or as dry vitamin E at levels of 100 to 800IU/day.
- Vitamin K as dry vitamin K at levels of 120 to 450mcg/day.
- Vitamin D as dry vitamin D, preferably as D3, at levels of 800 to 2000 IU/day. Vitamin D needs vary greatly depending on where people live geographically and how much time they spend outdoors. Some patients may need higher baseline levels depending on skin color, geographic area of residence, and lifestyle.
- After 3 to 6 months, patients can usually switch to tablets or capsules if they desire. Some find that chewable products remain the better option due to the number of pills or difficulty with swallowed forms.
- Some programs also advise additional magnesium, potassium, and zinc after this procedure.

## GOING BEYOND

If you have read this book, you now know there is a lot of gray area in nutrition. The recommended daily allowances (RDA) are mostly set based on levels of nutrients that keep most people from developing deficiency-based illnesses. They are not designed for people with chronic disease, malabsorption, or those who are interested in whether nutrition can actually advance health, not just prevent problems. If you compare the RDA for most nutrients to the UL, you will find that for many there is a pretty big gap. For some nutrients (e.g., B12), many believe they are safe even at thousands of times above the RDA. I only advise that if you do establish protocols that call for supraphysiological levels of nutrition, that you do so with a plan. Track what you do and follow your patients with labs. If you find success or if you find problems, share it with the community. The best way for us to advance our knowledge of nutrition and WLS is by the community working together to build data that supports what we do. This will benefit clinicians and patients alike.

## CONCLUSIONS

The best overall strategies for risk reduction are those that give clear instructions, both for products and follow-up. Patients will take nutrition more seriously if it is presented to them in a serious manner. The suggestions provided here are general rules that can be used to create your own guidelines. I hope that as our industry matures, we will come closer to agreement and be able to develop a true standard of care for nutrition after WLS. For now, combining baseline recommendations with regular follow-up is the best strategy for assuring long-term nutritional health of WLS patients.

# Final Thoughts

*Health is worth more than learning.*
**—Thomas Jefferson**

L ast night I was at a support group answering nutrition questions. One attendee asked me a touching question. He noted that when he first had surgery, his doctor had asked him to take calcium carbonate. Then, maybe a year later, his doctor told him they were now asking their patients to take calcium citrate because they had learned that this was better.

"Are we just an experiment?" he asked me.

There is no easy answer to this question. The fact is that we still have a lot to learn about normal human nutrition. We know more about how virtually every drug is digested, absorbed, and metabolized than we do about most of the nutrients that are essential to human life. Throw surgical malabsorption into the mix and we know a lot less. Add any chronic disease—diabetes, hypertension, asthma, even obesity itself—and we know less still.

So, yes, we are learning as we go. In reality, we are probably learning some lessons about normal human nutrition from weight loss surgery (WLS) patients. Hopefully, the lessons we learn will lead to better techniques and better strategies for preventing nutritional problems after surgery. Perhaps we will learn ways to refine surgical techniques so that patients still effectively lose weight without losing so much nutrition. Maybe we will develop elegant new techniques for delivering nutrients that overcome the hurdles of malabsorption. Possibly we will end up learning some keys to human nutrition that benefit people in far reaching corners of the world.

My hope, ultimately, is that we work together as a community toward a goal of healthy patients. Many of those undergoing surgery for obesity have never had a genuine vision of vital health. They have thought about not being sick, about not feeling pain, or about not being overweight. After surgery, there is a renewed chance for patients to experience a level of health they have not had in years or ever. Good nutrition and nutritional care provide excellent opportunities for patients to move beyond the place of being not sick to a new place of being truly healthy.

# PART 4:
# Appendices

## APPENDIX A—GUIDELINES FOR A GOOD MULTIVITAMIN (ADJUSTABLE GASTRIC BANDING [AGB] AND ROUX-EN-Y [RNY])

There are hundreds of multivitamin preparations on the market. The following are some general rules for selection:

1.   It should provide 100 to 300 percent of the daily value of the following: B2, B3 (niacin), B5 (pantothenic acid), folate, and biotin.

2.   It is best if multivitamins for RNY patients can provide at least 200 percent of the DV for thiamine (B1).

3.   It should provide at least 50mcg of B12.

4.   It is best if it also contains the accessory B vitamins choline and inositol.

5.   It should provide 30 to 200IU of vitamin E in its natural form. The natural forms of vitamin E are listed as "d," such as d-alpha tocopheryl acetate or succinate. If the form is preceded by "dl" then it is synthetic. You may need to look in the total ingredient listing to see this information.

6.   It should provide 100 to 200 percent of the DV of vitamin A, with no more than 5000IU coming from retinol (preformed vitamin A).

7.   It should provide between 400 and 600IU of vitamin D, and between 60 and 500mg of vitamin C.

8.   Vitamin K is optional and should be avoided in a supplement if patients are on blood thinners.

9.   It is best to have 100 percent of the DV for the following trace elements: Zinc, selenium, copper, manganese, chromium, and molybdenum. Look at the forms of the minerals carefully. If this is for a RNY patient, are they compatible with malabsorption? Most are best as chelates; selenium is best as selenomethionine.

10.  Fluoride, sodium, potassium, and phosphorus are best supplemented separately if needed and are not standard.

11.  Ultratrace elements, such as cobalt and nickel, are not necessary.

12.  There should be some calcium and magnesium. If you are not recommending separate calcium, pay close attention to how much the multivitamin provides. Calcium should be as a citrate for RNY patients. AGB patients should be able to tolerate most forms of calcium.

13. Iron is not always included in a multivitamin. If it is included, it should be present at the approximate daily value.

14. Iodine is optional. It is often left out of multivitamins due to possible allergic reactions and the prevalence of thyroid disease.

15. Look at what else is included. Are there other nutrients? Are there herbs? Antioxidants? Some of these can be nice additions, while others (such as some herbs) may pose an unnecessary risk. If you don't know what an ingredients is or why it is there, ask.

16. Read the fine print. Look at the "Other Ingredients" list. This is a long list of everything that goes into the product. This list should disclose everything, including non-nutritional ingredients. Look closely for ingredients that your patients may not tolerate, like sugar, lactose, or gluten.

17. Look at the allergen disclosure. This should be on the left side of the label and will tell you what, if any, common allergens are present in the product.

18. Finally, look for contact information. Product labels should contain an address and phone number. There should be someone you can call to ask questions, report problems, and get information.

**Additional considerations—Biliopancreatic diversion (BPD) and duodenal switch (DS).** Patients who have undergone BPD or DS or distal RNY patients who have more malabsorption may need some additional nutrients in their multivitamin, primarily higher doses of the fat-soluble vitamin A, E, D, and K. Again, it is not really known what levels are protective. The following ranges are considered safe in non-pregnant women and men. Women who are pregnant or plan to get pregnant should consult both with their bariatric program and their OB-GYN to discuss issues such as vitamin A and pregnancy. BPD/DS patients should consider the following:

1. Fat-soluble vitamins in formulas for BPD/DS patients should be in their dry, water-miscible forms.
2. Vitamin A (as retinol, not beta-carotene) should be in the range of 10,000 to 30,000IU.
3. Vitamin D should be in the range of 800 to 2000IU (but can be up to 10,000 for prevention).
4. Vitamin E should be in the range of 100 to 800IU.
5. Vitamin K should be in the range of 120 to 450mcg.

# APPENDIX B—PROFESSIONAL'S GUIDE TO NUTRITIONAL SUPPLEMENTS: UNDERSTANDING QUALITY AND REGULATORY ISSUES

Most weight loss surgery (WLS) programs in the United States recommend dietary supplements as part of their aftercare program. Health professionals are often confused about the regulatory and quality issues in the dietary supplement industry, which may lead to difficulty in evaluation of what products are safest and most reliable to recommend for patients with malabsorption. This appendix reviews the current regulatory status of dietary supplements in the United States in an effort to help clinicians better evaluate products they recommend for their patients.

**What is a dietary supplement?** It helps to start by understanding what a dietary supplement is and is not. Dietary supplements were defined in 1994 by Congress under the Dietary Supplement Health and Education Act (DSHEA). Under DSHEA, a product is a dietary supplement if it does the following:

1. Intended to supplement the diet
2. Contains dietary ingredients, such as vitamins, minerals, herbs (other than tobacco), amino acids, other natural substances, and/or their constituents
3. Ingested orally in the form of a pill, capsule, tablet, or liquid
4. Labeled on the front panel of the product as a dietary supplement
5. Sold and marketed as a dietary ingredient before October 15, 1994, or has been approved by the FDA as a new dietary ingredient (NDI)
6. Intended use is as a dietary supplement, not as a food or a drug.

**Supplement or drug?** Some substances are sold as both supplements and drugs. For vitamins, minerals, herbs, or other natural dietary ingredients, the intended use, language used to describe the product, or route of administration can be the defining point. Per the FDA, dietary supplements may not be used to or claim to diagnose, cure, mitigate, treat, or prevent a disease; substances that do this, or claim to do so, are drugs.

Niacin is a great example of a nutrient that is both a drug and a dietary supplement depending on the language used to describe it. Niacin is available both as a prescription drug and as a dietary supplement. For niacin products (such as Niaspan®) that are approved as drugs, companies may state that niacin can improve cholesterol and lower triglyceride levels. For niacin products sold as dietary supplements, companies may state that niacin supports a healthy cardiovascular system or helps to maintain cholesterol levels that are already within the normal ranges. It is not allowable for the supplement companies to discuss the ability of niacin to alter cholesterol and triglycerides, despite this being an established drug activity; they must stick to structure-function claims (see below). If a supplement company states that their niacin lowers cholesterol, it then becomes an unlicensed drug and the company may be subjected to fines or other penalties.

Route of delivery can also turn a dietary supplement into a drug. As stated above, dietary supplements must be orally ingested as pills, capsules, tablets, or liquids. They cannot be sprayed into or on the body; they cannot be applied as a cream, gel, or patch; they cannot be inhaled, sprayed into the nose, or dropped into the eyes; and they cannot be injected subcutaneously, intramuscularly, or intravenously. Substances delivered by these methods, without exception, are drugs, not dietary supplements.

**What is a medical food?** A lesser used category of natural products are those considered by the FDA to be medical foods. Medical foods are technically regulated under the Orphan Drug Act, not DSHEA. This means that they are not dietary supplements. Medical foods are defined as specialized dietary products that are not available for sale to the general public and must be supervised by a physician. (Some, however, are now being sold in pharmacies, and infant formulas—which are technically medical foods—are sold in mass retail.) The intent of medical foods is to manage a specific disease or condition. They must also meet the following criteria:

1.  They are intended to be used in patients who, "because of therapeutic or chronic medical needs have limited or impaired capacity to ingest, digest, absorb, or metabolize ordinary foodstuffs or certain nutrients, or who has other special medically determined nutrient requirements, the dietary management of which cannot be achieved by the modification of the normal diet alone."
2.  They are formulated for the partial or exclusive feeding of these patients, whether by oral intake or use with a feeding tube.
3.  They provide nutritional support for unique needs created by a unique medical condition.
4.  They are intended to be used only under medical supervision by patients requiring ongoing care that includes instruction on use of the product.

An example of a medical food would be phenylalanine-free foods for people with phenylketonuria (PKU) or gluten-free foods for those with celiac disease. At this point in time, there is very little FDA oversight of these products and associated claims, and most people in the dietary supplement industry consider this to be an enormous loophole in the FDA regulation of natural products. Unscrupulous companies see this as a way to sell products using drug claims that are not allowed under DSHEA and still avoid oversight. Like dietary supplements, it is not necessary for medical foods to be submitted to the FDA for approval prior to sale. Unlike dietary supplements, they may claim to treat or assist with disease states. Medical foods are also exempted from the Nutrition Labeling and Education Act (NLEA) that governs claims on food ingredients. Most industry experts consider it likely that the FDA will begin stricter oversight of medical foods in the near future. For the time being, however, while this law allows for the development of much needed dietary products for individuals with rare disorders and special needs, it also permits products that should be dietary supplements or drugs to come to market without much, if any, regulation.

**Who regulates products and the industry?** There is a general misconception that there is no federal agency with authority over the dietary supplement industry. In fact, the FDA has always had this authority, but the degree to which they have exercised it has changed much over the years. The FDA has had official authority over dietary ingredients since the passage of the 1938 Food, Drug, and Cosmetic Act. The 1994 passage of DSHEA merely created a new category and specific regulations for the industry to separate it from both foods and drugs.

**Manufacturing oversight.** The question of manufacturing quality and oversight for dietary supplements has been one of much debate both inside and outside of the industry. DSHEA authorized (but did not require) the FDA to create Good Manufacturing Practice (GMP) guidelines as it has in the past for the pharmaceutical industry. This was largely ignored for the better part of a decade. In the ensuing years, companies were required, as they had been for decades, to comply with food GMPs that essentially govern safety and sanitation. Industry groups, such as the National Nutritional Foods Association, created their own GMPs and associated certifications to help those who wished to comply with some standard. Some manufacturing facilities attained or retained status as OTC drug manufacturers, subjecting themselves to FDA GMP audits, but since none of these things were required, oversight was inconsistent at best.

In recent years, high-profile industry issues like use of hormone precursors and the ephedra recall focused increasing attention on regulation and safety, and many began to ask why the FDA had not exercised the right to implement GMPs. In 2003, under pressure from the government, the medical community, and the public over concerns about dietary supplement safety, the FDA proposed GMPs for the industry. Over the past two years, they have been reviewed, revised, caught in a tangle of politics on both sides of the issue, and ultimately submitted for a final approval by the Office of Management and Budget in October, 2005. In anticipation of the federal GMPs, many companies have taken this two-year period to bring up their standards. Unfortunately, as of the writing of this book, the finally ruling has still not been published, and GMPs continue to hang in limbo.

Ultimately, when they exist, the federal GMPs will regulate the activities of manufacturing, packaging, holding, and distributing of dietary ingredients and dietary supplements in a manner that assures that products cannot be adulterated or misbranded. They will further require manufacturers to evaluate the identity, purity, quality, strength, and composition of their dietary ingredients and dietary supplements by means similar to those required for the pharmaceutical industry. In their review of the industry prior to publication of proposed GMPs, the FDA noted multiple issues of concern, including substitution of incorrect ingredients (in some cases dangerous); use of non-food grade ingredients and chemicals in manufacture; product contamination with organisms such as *Klebsiella pneumonia* or botulism; contamination with lead and glass; unsafe and unsanitary manufacturing conditions; products containing levels of nutrients that do not match label claims; undeclared ingredients, such as potentially harmful allergens; lot-to-lot variability in product consistency; and other problems. It the hope of both the FDA and industry leaders that the enactment of GMPs will bring safety and quality to all areas of the industry, allowing for a significantly increased confidence in natural products.

It will still take some time once GMPs are finalized for companies around the country to either "comply or die." From the time of this publication, large firms will have one year and small firms will have three years to come into compliance. Until this time, the burden is still with the consumer to determine how a product is manufactured. Certification by an independent organization, such as NNFA or USP, or over-the-counter (OTC) certification is a good indication of a high standard in manufacture. Both NNFA and USP list on their websites companies who have voluntarily submitted to and passed GMP audits.

Those who wish to read the entire proposed federal GMPs can do so at the FDA website: http://www.cfsan.fda.gov/~dms/supplmnt.html

**Product oversight.** The FDA requires drugs to undergo premarket studies to establish safety, efficacy, dosing, interactions, and other specified parameters before their products are approved for sale. No such testing and approval is required for dietary supplements. However, the FDA does have oversight over manufacture, labeling, claims, and safety of dietary supplements.

As far as safety goes, the FDA currently treats dietary supplements more like foods than drugs. This means that companies selling dietary supplements are responsible for their safety, and the FDA is responsible for demonstrating that a product is unsafe before it can restrict use or recall the product from the market. It is currently not required for manufacturers or distributors of dietary supplements to collect or report adverse events to the FDA. Consumers or health professionals can file voluntary Adverse Event Reports (AERs) through Med Watch (www.fda.gov/medwatch).

The FDA regulates labeling for dietary supplements as it does for foods. Since the passage of DSHEA, the FDA has operated the Office of Nutritional Products, Labeling, and Dietary Supplements through the Center for Food Safety and Applied Nutrition (CFSAN). The FDA cites the purpose of this office as "monitoring safety, e.g., voluntary dietary supplement adverse event reporting, and product information, such as labeling, claims, package inserts, and accompanying literature." It has been the role of this office to attempt to clarify and make uniform the manner in which companies manufacturing and distributing supplements communicate to the public. Additionally, there has been increasing regulation of the way label information is conveyed (in the hopes of making it easier for consumers to understand), as well as requirements for full ingredient disclosure (including excipients, binders, fillers, encapsulating and coating materials, and allergens).

**Advertising and claims.** The FDA and the US Federal Trade Commission (FTC) technically work together to regulate what is said about dietary supplements. Where the FDA has primary jurisdiction over things that are on the product—the label, the packaging, inserts, and appended literature—the FTC has oversight over commercials, internet marketing, print media, catalogs, and direct marketing materials.

**Product claims.** The issue of claims made about dietary supplements is perhaps most irritating to physicians and confusing to consumers. As discussed above, the FDA and the FTC both have some oversight over claims, packaging, and label information. However, it seems that between these two agencies, they still struggle to maintain control over inconsistent, unproven, and just plain false information being distributed to consumers. This problem clearly has been compounded by the internet, which we now know is used by approximately 16 percent of the US adult population to seek out information on health. In the September 17, 2003, issue of *Journal of the American Medical Society*, Morris and Avorn conducted a survey of health claims made on the internet about the most common dietary supplements. The reviewers looked at 443 websites and applied FDA criteria to classify claims as "disease" or "non-disease" in nature. Of the surveyed sites, 76 percent were retail sites either selling product or directly linked to a vendor. Of this 76 percent, 81 percent (338 sites) made one or more health claims, with 55 percent of these claiming to treat, prevent, diagnose, or cure specific diseases. Moreover, 52 percent of retail sites failed to include the mandated federal disclaimer for dietary supplement sales. Only 12 percent of sites provided any reference materials to support claims. Thus, the authors concluded that despite supposed FTC authority to regulate these materials, the current enforcement of claims (at least on the internet) is quite poor and likely to mislead consumers.

By law, allowable claims for dietary supplement are supposed to meet both FDA and FTC criteria. The FDA offers general guidelines for structure-function claims, language for approved health claims (very limited), and required disclaimers (such as those that caution use in pregnancy and nursing). The FTC further offers guidelines for advertising that are designed to assure that materials are truthful and not misleading in nature. They further require claims to be adequately substantiated by solid scientific data.

Details of what the FDA requires can be accessed at http://www.cfsan.fda.gov/~dms/ds-labl.html; FTC requirements are available at http://www.ftc.gov/bcp/conline/pubs/buspubs/dietsupp.htm.

It may be easiest to understand the difficulty with these regulations by exploring real examples. Calcium is a nutrient that works well for this purpose. Most of us would be likely to agree that calcium is an important part of strong bones and that adequate intake helps to prevent, and perhaps even treat, bone loss. The FDA allows the nutritional supplement industry to use the following claim:

"Regular exercise and a healthy diet with enough calcium helps teens and young adult white and Asian women maintain good bone health and may reduce their high risk of osteoporosis later in life."

Many nutritional companies have shunned this allowable claim due to its restrictive nature and have instead chosen to use structure-function language that might read something like: "Calcium helps to support healthy teeth and bones."

Still other companies may ignore all guidelines and opt to make claims that calcium, or their calcium in particular, prevents osteoporosis or even that it treats or prevents a broad range of other conditions, such as cancer or diabetes.

Another good example is niacin (B3). For niacin products that are licensed as drugs, companies may state that niacin can improve cholesterol and lower triglyceride levels. For niacin products sold as dietary supplements, companies may state that niacin supports a healthy cardiovascular system. It is not allowable for the supplement companies to discuss the ability of niacin to alter cholesterol and triglycerides, despite this being an established drug activity; they must stick to structure-function claims. If a supplement company states that their niacin lowers cholesterol, it then becomes an unlicensed drug and the company may be subjected to fines or other punishment.

Bariatric professionals should also be aware that the FTC has placed specific emphasis on products and companies that market products for weight loss. Following a 2002 FTC report that found more than half of the advertising for products and services for weight loss contained false or unsubstantiated claims, the FTC began increasing oversight specifically targeted at this industry segment. In 2003, the FTC began a campaign called "Red Flag," which gave guidelines to media on how to spot false advertising of weight loss products. Subsequently in 2004, they launched "Operation Big Fat Lie," which levied aggressive fines against some of the biggest companies with misleading advertising. Still, not all companies comply with advertising rules, and many of these companies are starting to see both pre- and postoperative weight loss surgery patients as a rich source of revenue. Patients should be counseled on what products are both safe and effective to use both before and after surgery. Health professionals may additionally want to advise them of how to spot false claims. This information can be viewed on the FTC web site at: http://www.ftc.gov/bcp/menu-health.htm, under the "Business Information" section.

My general advice to health professionals and patients alike is that claims for a product should not be taken at face value, companies should be able to produce substantiation to support any claims made, and that if it sounds too good to be true it probably is!

**Quality of ingredients.** Ingredients in dietary supplements—from vitamins to herbs—come from all over the world. While some ingredients are domestic, many come from China, India, and third-world nations where controls on processing may not match those in the US or Europe. Again, the new manufacturing GMPs will help to diminish or eliminate the use of questionably sourced raw materials in manufacture by requiring more independent testing of raw materials, microbial screening, quarantine, and other quality controls. Many manufacturers currently rely on the certificate of analysis (C of A) provided by the supplier to be truthful and accurate. Select manufacturers and those preparing for GMPs may use in-house or outsourced laboratory analysis to verify materials.

Manufacturers can choose from a variety of sources, forms, and grades of nutrients. The current accepted standards for most nutrients follow the guidelines set out by the United States Pharmacopoeia (USP) and National Formulary (NF). These standards exist for over 2000 ingredients. The FCC (Food Chemical Codex) writes standards for substances commonly used as excipients. All of these designators (USP, NF, FCC) may appear on labels of products if manufacturers and distributors choose to indicate that they are using certified ingredients, although they are often omitted due to space limitations. For some ingredients, especially herbs, there may be no standard set, and it is harder to judge from a label the quality of the ingredients. Additionally, some manufacturers may not supply this information on the label and it is then the responsibility of the consumer obtain it.

**Nutrient forms.** Both in nature and in supplements, nutrients can be present in a variety of forms. Some of these forms may have different activities in the body, may be more or less bioavailable, or may even have different levels of toxicity. Again, niacin makes a great example. Niacin is commonly found in two forms: Niacin (nicotinic acid) and niacinamide (nicotinamide). Both of these substances are classified as niacin and vitamin B3, and are utilized in the body to form coenzymes. However, there are vital differences in their functions. The acid form is the only form demonstrated to lower cholesterol and triglycerides; it also causes flushing. The amide form will not lower blood fats or cause flushing. Since the amide form is most common in dietary supplements, physicians recommending OTC niacin for cardiovascular health would need to specify this for patients. All prescription forms of niacin use the acid form for this reason.

Another excellent example is vitamin E. The most common form of vitamin E found in nutritional supplements is synthetic dl-alpha-tocopherol (all-rac-alpha- tocopherol). Because one isomer making up half the mix is not usable by the human body, this form is not nearly as bioavailable as natural vitamin E. The natural form, d-alpha-tocopherol or RRR-alpha-tocopherol, is almost twice as bioavailable and is thus much preferred. Still, since consumers may not be familiar with the complex nomenclature, they may think that they are getting a high level of vitamin E in a product that really only provides half the labeled amount in a useful form. Similar examples can be seen for many vitamins and minerals, including calcium, iron, selenium, and thiamine.

**Chew, swallow, or drink?** There are also many choices for how products are delivered. The most common forms are chewable tablets, liquids, hard-coated tablets, and gelatin capsules. Regardless of the way a product is delivered to the body, the quality of the ingredients is still of great importance. Despite what a manufacturer may say, merely putting something into a liquid medium does not give it 100-percent bioavailability—it just eliminates one level of work the body would have to do to break the product apart. The form of the nutrient itself, amount delivered, nutritional status at the time of delivery, and other factors all play into bioavailability, so nothing is ever 100 percent. Hard-coated tablets pose the greatest potential challenge to WLS patients. Most of these preparations are designed to break apart with stomach acid and churning. Some will break apart without this, but it's hard to know which ones. If you have a tried and true product in a coated tablet that you use, there is no need to change, but if patients are going on their own to find one at the store, it is probably not the best choice. Two-piece gelatin capsules are a great choice as they will break apart with moisture and heat and require no mechanics. Chewable products that are broken apart with the teeth and liquids can also be good choices so long as the ingredients are appropriate for WLS patients. With liquids, stability can be an issue and they should always be checked for an expiration stamp. Products with crystal formation or a lot of sediment should be suspect. The delivery system that you choose can also help with patient adherence. You may have a product you love, but if your patient can't swallow it or despises the taste, he or she is not likely to stick with your recommendation.

**Excipients, binders, fillers, and "other ingredients."** All dietary supplements contain other ingredients that are not active constituents in the product. These may include binding agents, flow agents, fillers, coating material, disintegrants, lubricants, granulating agents, colors, sweeteners, and in addition, it is common for these raw materials to include one or more additives themselves. For example, very small nutrients like folic acid are diluted to make them easier to mix and measure. Common diluting agents include calcium and lactose. Fat-soluble vitamins that have undergone an oil-to-powder process to make them compressible and more bioavailable may have multiple additives, such as calcium, silicon dioxide, lactose, starch, gelatin, vitamin E, and preservatives. All ingredients, including those pre-mixed with raw materials, should be declared on the label of a product below the Supplement Facts box on the right panel. New allergen disclosure regulations that became active on January 1, 2006, require manufacturers to obtain allergen declarations from all raw material suppliers and properly disclaim allergens on product labels. Consumers with known allergens should be advised to closely read labels for this type of information, and would be wise to call the manufacturer if there are any questions.

**Conclusions.** The dietary supplement industry is currently in a state of maturing. While regulations do exist and more are on the way, the problem of enforcement still looms large and makes it difficult for both consumers and medical professionals to evaluate key issues related to safety and efficacy. For now, the best assurance that physicians have if they recommend dietary supplements is to seek out products from manufacturers that have been GMP-certified by an independent auditor or by the FTC as an OTC drug manufacturer. In regards to advertising, it is important for physicians to recognize that their patients are likely to encounter many fraudulent or unsubstantiated claims when they investigate dietary supplements, and that they as health experts may be called upon to comment on these issues. Health professionals too should be aware that claims about products may not be backed by science that has been reviewed by any authority, and should take care to assess the science themselves before taking claims at face value.

As the industry of bariatric surgery continues to grow, the dietary supplement industry will focus more on these patients as a specific and potentially lucrative market. Helping patients to understand these issues is important to their long-term health, as well as to the long-term success of the WLS industry. The healthier patients are, the better it is for everyone. Clinicians working with bariatric surgery patients need to learn exactly what their patients are taking, encourage open lines of communication, seek information from product companies, and establish nutrition protocols that are based on sound recommendations.

## Resources

*FTC Guidance Documents for Consumers and Businesses:* http://www.ftc.gov/bcp/menu-health.htm

*FTC Diet and Fitness Center:* http://www.ftc.gov/dietfit/

*FDA Center for Food Safety and Applied Nutrition:* http://www.cfsan.fda.gov/

*FDA Office of Nutritional Products, Labeling, and Dietary Supplements:* http://www.cfsan.fda.gov/~dms/onplds.html

*FDA Med Watch Program:* http://www.fda.gov/medwatch/

*National Institutes of Health Office of Dietary Supplements:* http://ods.od.nih.gov/

*National Nutritional Foods Association* (offering both GMP certification and product testing programs since 1999): http://www.nnfa.org

*NSF International* (offers GMP certification, ISO certification, ingredient validation services to the dietary supplement industry since 2003): http://www.nsf.org

*United States Pharmacopeia* (Offers the USP Verified program for both ingredients and manufacturing): http://www.usp.org

*A new dietary ingredient (NDI)* is a vitamin, mineral, herb, amino acid, or a concentrate, metabolite, constituent, extract, or combination of any of the above dietary ingredients that was not marketed in the United States as a dietary supplement prior to October 15, 1994. These substances must be submitted to the FDA for approval a minimum of 75 days before they are made available for sale.

*Medical Foods.* US Food and Drug Administration, Center for Food Safety and Applied Nutrition. Available at: http://vm.cfsan.fda.gov/~dms/ds-medfd.html. Accessed December 20, 2005.

Tu HT, Hargraves JL. Seeking health care information: Most consumers still on the sidelines. *HSC Alerts* 2003;Issue Brief No. 61. Available at: http://www.hschange.org/index.cgi?topic=topic03 Access date: December 3, 2005.

Morris CA, Avorn J. Internet marketing of herbal products. *JAMA* 2003;290:1505–9.

The disclaimer is as follows: This (these) statement(s) has(have) not been evaluated by the Food and Drug Administration. This (these) product(s) is(are) not intended to diagnose, treat, cure, or prevent any disease.

US Food and Drug Administration. Center for Food Safety and Applied Nutrition. A Food Labeling Guide. Sept 1994 (Ed rev Jun 1999, Nov 2000). Accessed 12 Dec 2005. http://www.cfsan.fda.gov/~dms/flg-6c.html

Traber MG, Elsner A, Brigelius-Flohe R. Synthetic as compared with natural vitamin E is preferentially excreted as alpha-CEHC in human urine: Studies using deuterated alpha-tocopheryl acetates. *FEBS Lett* 1998;437(1-2):145–8.

## APPENDIX C—BASIC MICRONUTRIENT LAB TESTS AFTER WEIGHT LOSS SURGERY

- **1 Month**
  - Thiamine if there is vomiting or symptoms

- **3 Months**
  - Thiamine if there is vomiting or symptoms
  - Metabolic panel with PTH, and electrolytes including calcium

- **6 Months**
  - Thiamine if there is vomiting or symptoms
  - Metabolic panel with PTH, and electrolytes including calcium
  - Serum B12, iron indices
  - Prealbumin

- **12 Months**
  - Thiamine if there is vomiting or symptoms
  - Metabolic panel with PTH, and electrolytes including calcium
  - Serum B12, iron indices
  - Folate, homocysteine
  - Prealbumin
  - 25-OH D
  - If duodenal switch (DS), add vitamin A and zinc

- **Annually**
  - Metabolic panel with PTH, and electrolytes including calcium
  - Serum B12, iron indices
  - Folate, homocysteine
  - Prealbumin
  - 25-OH D
  - If DS, add vitamin A and zinc
  - Review symptoms and determine if additional tests are indicated

- **18 to 24 Months**
  - DEXA or other evaluation of bone density
  - This should be repeated as results indicate

# APPENDIX D—DEFICIENCIES CAUSING VARIOUS MEDICAL CONDITIONS

## Deficiencies causing anemia
- Iron
  - Type: Microcytic, hypochromic
- Copper
  - Type: Microcytic, hypochromic
- Zinc
- B12
  - Type: Macrocytic
- Folate
  - Type: Macrocytic

- Vitamin C
  - Type: Microcytic—due to secondary iron deficiency

### Deficiencies causing neuropathy
*Common*
- B12
- Thiamine
  - Hallmarks:
      Burning dysesthesia
      Weakness
      Muscle loss, distal wasting
      Trophic changes
      Graded sensory loss
      Pain and heaviness in the extremities
      Tibial edema
      Glove and stocking neuropathy
      Difficulty climbing and standing

*Less Common*
- Niacin
  - Hallmarks:
      Sensory neuropathy with itching and burning in the hands and feet
      Sensory excitation
      Cold-seeking behavior (i.e., patients desire cold baths)
      Tremor
- B6
- B5
- Vitamin E
- Copper—can look just like B12 deficiency

### Deficiencies causing hair loss
- Iron
- Zinc
- Protein

## APPENDIX E—NUTRITIONAL CAUSES OF HAIR LOSS

A common fear and complaint of bariatric surgery patients is postoperative hair loss. The most common type of hair loss after weight loss surgery is a diffuse loss known as telogen effluvium, which can have both nutritional and non-nutritional causes.

Human hair follicles have two states: anagen, a growth phase; and telogen, a dormant stage. All hairs begin their life in the anagen phase, grow for some period of time, then shift into the telogen phase, which lasts for about 100 to 120 days. Following this, the hair will fall out. Typically, about 90 percent of hairs are anagen and 10 percent are telogen at any given time.

Specific types of stressors can result of a shift in a much greater percentage of hairs into the telogen phase. The stressors known to result in telogen effluvium include: High fever, severe infection, major surgery, acute physical trauma, chronic debilitating illness (such as cancer or end-stage liver disease), hormonal disruption (such as pregnancy, childbirth, or discontinuation of estrogen therapy), acute weight loss, crash dieting, anorexia, low protein intake, iron or zinc deficiency, heavy metal toxicity, and some medications (such as beta-blockers, anticoagulants, retinoids, and immunizations).

Nutritional issues aside, weight loss surgery (WLS) patients already have two major risk factors for hair loss: Major surgery and rapid weight loss. These alone are likely to account for much of the hair loss seen after surgery. In the absence of a nutritional issue, hair loss will continue until all hairs that have shifted into telogen phase have fallen out. There is no way of switching them back to the anagen phase. Hair loss will rarely last for more than six months in the absence of a dietary cause. Because hair follicles are not damaged in telogen effluvium, hair should then regrow.

Discrete nutritional deficiencies are known to cause and contribute to telogen effluvium. One would be more suspicious of a nutritional contribution to post-WLS hair loss if:
1. Hair loss continued more than one year after surgery
2. Hair loss started more than six months after surgery
3. Patient has difficulty eating and/or has not adhered to supplementation
4. Patient has more rapid than expected weight loss
5. Other symptoms of deficiency are present.

**Iron.** Iron is the single nutrient most highly correlated with hair loss. The correlation between non-anemic iron deficiency and hair loss was first described in the early 1960s, although little to no follow-up research was conducted until this decade. While new research is conflicted as to the significance of ferritin as a diagnostic tool in alopecia, it has still been found that a significant number of people with telogen effluvium respond to iron therapy. Optimal iron indices for hair health have not been established, although there is some good evidence that a ferritin level below 40ug/L is highly associated with hair loss in women.[1]

**Zinc.** Zinc deficiency has been tied to hair loss in both animal studies and human cases. There is data linking zinc deficiency in humans to both telogen effluvium and immune-mediated hair loss. Zinc deficiency is not a well-recognized problem after any procedure other than duodenal switch (DS). Nonetheless, a group of researchers chose to study high-dose zinc supplementation as a therapeutic agent for WLS-related hair loss in patients with vertical banded gastroplasty (VBG).[2] The 1996 intervention trial administered 200mg of zinc sulfate (45mg elemental zinc) three times daily to postoperative patients with hair loss. This was in addition to the multivitamin and iron supplements that patients were already taking. No labs for zinc or other nutrients were conducted. Researchers found that in patients taking the zinc, 100 percent had cessation of hair loss after six months. In five patients, hair loss resumed after zinc was stopped and was arrested again with renewed supplementation. It is important to note that in telogen effluvium of non-nutritional origin, hair loss would be expected to stop normally within six months. In the absence of any laboratory studies, and with no placebo, the only patients of interest here are those who began to lose hair again after stopping zinc. Further study of this connection might be of value not only in examining the connection between zinc and hair, but (perhaps more importantly) examining zinc status in WLS patients.

The tolerable upper intake level (UL) for zinc is set at 40mg in adults. This study utilized a daily dose of more than three times that level. Not only can these levels cause gastrointestinal distress, but chronic toxicity (mostly associated with copper depletion) can start at levels of 60mg/day. Information related to this study has made its way to many a support group and chat room, even to doctors' offices, with the message of "high-dose zinc will prevent hair loss after WLS." Patients should be advised that high-dose zinc therapy is unproven and should only be done under supervision due to the associated risks of toxicity. For a more complete picture of zinc toxicity, see Chapter 13.

**Protein.** Low protein intake is associated with hair loss mostly through knowledge of protein-calorie malnutrition. Protein malnutrition has been reported with DS and in Roux-en-Y (RNY) surgery patients to a much lesser degree. Little is known about incidence, as only around eight percent of surgeons track lab screenings that measure total protein, albumen, or prealbumin.[3] Limited studies suggest that patients with the most rapid or greatest amounts of weight loss are at greatest risk.[4] With surgical reduction of the stomach, hydrochloric acid,[5] pepsinogen, and normal churning are all significantly reduced or eliminated. Furthermore, pancreatic enzymes that would also aid in protein digestion are redirected to a lower part of the small intestine. It is thus likely that maldigestion, rather than malabsorption, is responsible for most cases. Some studies have also implicated low protein intake.[6]

Research also indicates that low levels of the amino acid l-lysine are contributory to hair loss and that repletion of lysine stores may both improve iron status and improve hair regrowth. In a study of anemic patients with hair loss who were supplemented with 1.5 to 2 grams of l-lysine in addition to their iron therapy, ferritin levels increased more substantially over iron therapy alone.[7]

Many individuals believe that supplementing or topically applying the nutrient biotin will either help to prevent hair loss or will improve hair regrowth. To date, there is no science that would support either of these presumptions. While biotin deficiency can cause dermatitis, hair loss is only known to occur in experimentally induced states in animal models or in extreme cases of prolonged diets composed exclusively of egg whites.

**Other.** Other nutrients associated with hair health include vitamin A, inositol, folate, B-6, and essential fatty acids. Hair loss can also be caused by systemic diseases, including thyroid disease and PCOS, and is influenced by genetics.

**Conclusions.** Hair loss can be distressing to WLS patients, and many will try nutritional interventions themselves to see if they can prevent or mitigate it. Unfortunately, there is little evidence that early hair loss is preventable because it is mostly likely caused by surgery and rapid weight loss. Later hair loss, however, can be indicative of a nutritional problem, especially iron deficiency, and may be a clinically useful sign. Educating patients about the potential for hair loss and possible underlying causes can help them to make informed choices and avoid wasting money on gimmicks that may have little real value.

### References
1. Rushton DH. Nutritional factors and hair loss. *Clin Exp Dermatol* 2002;27(5):396–404.
2. Neve H, Bhatti W, Soulsby C, et al. Reversal of hair loss following vertical gastroplasty when treated with zinc sulphate. *Obes Surg* 1996;6(1):63–5.
3. Updegraff TA, Neufeld NJ. Protein, iron, and folate status of patients prior to and following surgery for morbid obesity. *J Am Diet Assoc* 1981;78(2):135–40.
4. Segal A, Kinoshita Kussunoki D, Larino MA. Postsurgical refusal to eat: Anorexia nervosa, bulimia nervosa, or a new eating disorder? A case series. *Obes Surg* 2004;14(3):353–360.
5. Behrns KE, Smith CD, Sarr MG. Prospective evaluation of gastric acid secretion and cobalamin absorption following gastric bypass

for clinically severe obesity. *Dig Dis Sci* 1994;39(2):315–20.

6.    Moize V, Geliebter A, Gluck ME, et al. Obese patients have inadequate protein intake related to protein intolerance up to 1 year following Roux-en-Y gastric bypass. *Obes Surg* 2003;13(1):23–8.

7.    Mock DM. Biotin. In: Shils M, Olson JA, Shike M, Ross AC (eds). *Nutrition in Health and Disease, Ninth Edition.* Baltimore, MD: Williams & Wilkins;1999:459–66.

# APPENDIX F—RESOURCES

## Textbooks on Nutrition

- *Modern Nutrition in Health and Disease, Ninth Edition* by Maurice E. Shils, James A. Olson, Moshe Shike, A. Catherine Ross (Editors). Lippincott Williams & Wilkins, 1999.
- *Advanced Nutrition and Human Metabolism, Fourth Edition* by Sareen S. Gropper, Jack L. Smith, and James L. Groff. Wadsworth Publishing, 2004.
- *Handbook of Clinical Nutrition, Third Edition* by Douglas C. Heimburger and Roland L. Weinsier. C.V. Mosby, 1997.
- *Biochemical, Physiological & Molecular Aspects of Human Nutrition, Second Edition* by Martha Stipanuk. W.B. Saunders Company, 2006.
- *Medical Nutrition from Marz, Second Edition* by Russell B. Marz. Omni-Press, 1997

## Internet Resources

- www.nutraingredients-usa.com—up-to-date nutrition research from around the world
- www.vitasearch.com—searchable database and newsletter with research summaries
- www.whfoods.com—Worlds Healthiest Foods—a great resource for food/nutrition information
- ods.od.nih.gov—Office of Dietary Supplements—From the National Institutes of Health
- www.nap.edu—National Academies Press—all the Dietary Reference Intakes, Food Chemical Codex, research, plus 29 other texts for free online
- www.umm.edu/altmed—University of Maryland Center for Integrative Medicine—comprehensive database for vitamins, herbs, interactions, nutrient depletion by drugs and more
- www.nutrition.org—*American Journal of Clinical Nutrition* and the *Journal of Nutrition*—most full content is free
- www.nutritionj.com—*Nutrition Journal*—free online journal form BioMedCentral
- www.merck.com—*Merck Manual* online